Infant-Toddler Assessment:
An Interdisciplinary Approach

Infant-Toddler Assessment:
An Interdisciplinary Approach

Louis M. Rossetti, Ph.D.
Associate Professor,
Department of Communicative Disorders,
University of Wisconsin–Oshkosh

8700 Shoal Creek Boulevard
Austin, Texas

Printed in the United States of America

Library of Congress Cataloging-in-Publication Data

Rossetti, Louis Michael.
    Infant-toddler assessment : an interdisciplinary approach / Louis
M. Rossetti.
        p.   cm.
    Reprint. Originally published: Boston : Little, Brown, c1990.
    Includes bibliographical references and index.
    ISBN 0-89079-312-3
    1. Child development—Research—Methodology.   2. Child psychology-
-Research—Methodology.   I. Title.
    [DNLM: 1. Child Development.   2. Child Psychology.   3. Data
Collection—methods.   WS 105.5.E8 R829i 1990a]
RJ131.R66   1991
618.92—dc20
DNLM/DLC
for Library of Congress   90-9185
                                                                          CIP

pro·ed

8700 Shoal Creek Boulevard
Austin, Texas 78758

1   2   3   4   5   6   7   8   9   10   95   94   93   92   91

This text is affectionately dedicated
to the six most important women in my life:
Elizabeth, Robyn, Nicole, Jennifer, Bethany,
and my wife Ruth,
without whose constant encouragement and
support it would never have been completed.

Contents

Preface   **ix**

Acknowledgments   **xi**

Chapter 1.   The Case for Infant-Toddler Assessment   **1**

Chapter 2.   Recipients of Infant-Toddler Assessment   **25**

Chapter 3.   Models for Infant-Toddler Assessment   **55**

Chapter 4.   General and Specific Assessment   **87**
                  Considerations

Chapter 5.   Collecting and Reporting Assessment Data   **119**

Chapter 6.   Specific Assessment Domains and Procedures   **141**

Chapter 7.   Pulling It All Together   **209**

Appendix A.   Sample Questionnaires   **233**

Appendix B.   Annotated Bibliography of Infant and Child   **255**
                  Assessment Instruments

Index   **285**

Preface

Several problems face practitioners who provide services to children who are developmentally delayed or at risk of being so. First, there are few courses on infant-toddler assessment. Second, there are not many textbooks designed to equip practitioners with the skills necessary to provide accurate assessment of infants and toddlers. As a result, those now involved in assessment activity have had to equip themselves, often through trial and error, to gain expertise in assessment. Third, misconceptions about the process of infant-toddler assessment, the purposes it fulfills, and its inherent limitations further frustrate practitioners. These problems will intensify as federal legislation mandates the provision of services — both identification and intervention — to infants and toddlers in the 1990s.

The purpose of this text, in light of the problems and frustrations experienced by practitioners involved in infant-toddler assessment, is to identify the important issues and to provide direction in dealing with the frustrations. Topics covered include an overall philosophy of assessment; the purposes of assessing infants and toddlers; the recipients of assessment activity; models of service delivery; when to initiate assessment activity; the developmental domains to be assessed; what to consider when choosing assessment instruments; legislation on services provided for children 0 to 5 years of age; personnel training issues; and coordinating the results of assessment information and effectively communicating with other professionals.

As an increasing number of professionals from a wide array of disciplines become involved and interested in issues related to infant-toddler assessment, a text of this nature is needed. These issues include measuring program effectiveness, monitoring developmental progress, validating assessment instruments, and making programming and intervention decisions. The intended audience for this text consists of professionals from a variety of academic disciplines who share the common goal of obtaining accurate and reliable information on infant-toddler developmental skill mastery. This text is directed toward furthering the mutual achievement of that goal.

L.M.R.

Acknowledgments

I have been fortunate to have the opportunity to work with College-Hill Press a second time. Once again I have found College-Hill to be interested first and foremost in quality publications. This attitude is reflected in the way they deal with authors, the process of publication, and the quality of the books published. Although the second time around I was more familiar with the overall process of writing a text, College-Hill consistently provided the support and encouragement that I needed at the right time. Many thanks to Marie Linvill and the entire College-Hill staff.

Many thanks also to Lee Snyder-McLean. Lee's familiarity with child development, both as a researcher and a clinician, has made her once again the ideal editor for me to work with. Her familiarity with the writing process, her constant encouragement, and her timely reminders to keep the process going were just what I needed.

I would also like to express appreciation to my colleagues in the Communicative Disorders Program at the University of Wisconsin-Oshkosh. They have been patient with me for the past 18 months during the completion of this text. I would in particular like to thank Jack Kile for his passion for the clinic. He stimulated my thinking in ways that he will never know. Janis Kuba also helped me think through various aspects of the assessment process. Her clinical insights were quite valuable to me. Hal Homann, Terry Monicken, Barbara Ansell, and Marie Rouse created an atmosphere in which increased attention toward writing could take place. Kathleen Robl, program secretary, made my job as coordinator easy. I am very appreciative of her support. I have received support from the entire university community, both faculty and administration, and for this I am truly grateful.

I would also like to thank a steady stream of bright, energetic, and talented graduate students at the University of Wisconsin-Oshkosh. It is simply not possible to become complacent when surrounded by graduate students who challenge faculty and make the learning process a mutual one. Finally, many friends, too numerous to mention, assisted me with their encouragement, support and, most important, prayers. I am forever indebted to them for the degree to which they cared for me just when I most needed it.

Infant-Toddler Assessment:
An Interdisciplinary Approach

CHAPTER 1

The Case for Infant-Toddler Assessment

Historical Considerations

Societal Factors

Impact of the Civil Rights Movement

Impact of the Media and Organized Support Groups

Research Activity
  Study of Normal Infant
    Development
  Study of the Efficacy of
    Early Intervention
  Study of the Parents' Role
    in Early Intervention

Federal Legislation
  P.L. 94-142: The Education
    of All Handicapped
    Children Act
  P.L. 99-457: Education of
    the Handicapped
    Amendments of 1986

Summary

Study Questions

References

HISTORICAL CONSIDERATIONS

Many types of professionals are interested in the delivery of assessment and intervention services to handicapped infants and toddlers. The increasing number of professions involved with this unique population has given rise to strategies that enable professionals to work together in providing such services. Models describing how professionals can better work together are available to all who are interested. This text has in large measure evolved from the realization that numerous people share a common goal: the delivery of high-quality services to handicapped or at-risk infants and toddlers (birth through 3 years of age) and their families. The information to follow is directed toward professionals from across disciplinary boundaries who share this common interest. Hence, this text is targeted toward those already providing such services or those who anticipate doing so in the near future.

Over the past 50 years a variety of forces have interacted advantageously to influence positively the status of infants and toddlers. These factors include (1) increased research activity related to normal infant development as well as investigations designed to assess the efficacy of early intervention with handicapped infants and toddlers; (2) social pressure to ensure equal rights for minorities, including the handicapped; (3) litigation to guarantee such rights; (4) state and federal mandates to expand educational opportunities for handicapped persons of all ages; (5) an awareness of the efficacious nature of early identification and treatment of persons with disabilities; and (6) multiple grass-roots efforts to demonstrate a more humanitarian posture toward persons with handicapping conditions. Because of the interaction of these forces, infants and toddlers with handicapping conditions may be identified early to ensure timely intervention. As a prelude to a discussion of the need to identify early those children who display developmental delay, material on the evolution of service provision for infants and toddlers will be presented. Each of the forces that has been identified as affecting services to infants and toddlers will be discussed.

SOCIETAL FACTORS

A powerful force that has exerted influence to enhance the status of infants and toddlers is reflected in societal awareness of and desire for optimal development for all persons. Historically, physically and behaviorally different offspring were treated quite differently than they are today. They were either killed outright or simply left to die (Filler, 1983). It was not until the eighteenth century that a more humanitarian philosophy began to prevail. At this time more systematic and formalized attempts to identify, treat, and care for persons who displayed physical and behavioral differences emerged, and a desire to understand the genesis of handicapping conditions from a rational standpoint came into being. Even in light of this more humanitarian view, efforts to treat and care for handicapped individuals were relatively rare. The nineteenth century witnessed improvements in overall conditions for mentally and physically handicapped persons. The primary orientation, however, was directed toward basic care.

The early twentieth century was not an optimistic time for the education of handicapped individuals. This state of affairs was due in large measure to the nativist view of intelligence. The nativists viewed intelligence as primarily determined by heredity and thus subject to only limited modification through educational intervention. As a result, the bulk of services to handicapped persons took the form of institutionalization. Large residential facilities for the deaf, blind, mentally retarded, emotionally disturbed, and any one of a number of other chronic conditions proliferated throughout the United States and Europe. Only a handful of states had special education classes, and their existence was voluntary rather than mandated by law. Over time, as a large and impressive body of information emerged pointing to the importance of the environment as a major factor in determining intelligence, a move away from institutionalization took place. This movement continues today.

IMPACT OF THE CIVIL RIGHTS MOVEMENT

Also during the early twentieth century, society in general became more concerned about minority groups' rights and welfare. Part of this awareness was directed toward handicapped persons. Many credit the Civil Rights movement for directing attention toward the rights of the handicapped. The Civil Rights movement of the early 1950s required that the nation face the active discriminatory acts perpetuated in training, hiring, housing, and the public schools for racial minorities, the poor, and the handicapped (Allen, 1984). The Civil Rights movement brought into sharp focus the rights of the individual and, in particular, the rights of children. Enhanced sensitivity resulted in litigation designed to secure the rights of minorities. It was in part through litigation of this nature that the current status of state and federal legislation dealing with service provision for handicapped persons came into being.

Several early court cases began to shape the status of educational practice regarding minorities and handicapped persons. One of these, *Brown vs. Board of Education* (1954), addressed the public schools' separate but equal stance. The outcome of this case ensured equal educational opportunities for all children attending public schools. It was a number of years, however, before equal educational opportunity was ensured for handicapped children.

In the early 1970s, advocacy efforts by parents helped to create state and federal legislation regarding educational services for handicapped children (Gallagher, 1984). Parents took their concerns for educational issues to court. In a series of cases throughout the 1970s, handicapped children's rights were affirmed to include:

A free and appropriate education
Due process for grievances
Special education services without regard to arguments about lack of funds
Freedom from being labeled handicapped or being placed in a special education program without an adequate diagnosis

IMPACT OF THE MEDIA AND
ORGANIZED SUPPORT GROUPS

These societal forces, which have significantly enhanced the status of handicapped persons, continue today. Print media and all other forms of mass communication have devoted increasing attention to the plight of all varieties of handicapping conditions across age groups. National organizations promote a vast array of concerns regarding a variety of handicapping conditions. These include, to mention only a few, organizations that educate the general public about the mentally retarded, educationally impaired, visually impaired, communicatively impaired, and sensory impaired as well as those individuals having specific medical disorders that result in handicapping conditions. Lobbying efforts continue on the state and federal level to promote the legal rights of persons with all types of handicaps. Prominent persons, including politicians and entertainment personalities, have throughout the 1970s and 1980s publicly promoted the rights of handicapped persons. One indication of the general public's interest in the status of handicapped persons has been the vast amounts of money raised on local, state, national, and international levels through grass-roots efforts as well as highly organized and sponsored fund-raising activities. Parents and family no longer shield a handicapped child from society. Instead, support groups made up of parents and other interested persons work to assist families in facing the unique set of challenges the handicapped person and the family face. Handicapped persons are increasingly viewed as valuable members of society and as individuals who are more like than unlike nonhandicapped persons.

RESEARCH ACTIVITY

STUDY OF NORMAL INFANT DEVELOPMENT

At the same time that society as a whole was changing its attitudes toward handicapped persons, researchers from a variety of disciplines were significantly expanding the base of knowledge regarding infant and toddler development. One of the primary forces that has given impetus to the present degree of interest focused on infants and toddlers has been an increase in research activity directed toward children 0 to 3 years of age.

In any field of endeavor, basic research serves to define more clearly and to explain the particular area under investigation. One of the outcomes of the activity directed towards infants and toddlers has been to ascribe to the infant abilities that were previously not thought to be innately present at birth. Hence, the concept of the competent infant evolved. The result was an increasingly sophisticated picture of infant and toddler abilities. Because of this intense scrutiny of infant and toddler abilities, a comprehensive and sometimes surprising picture of the inborn capabilities of infants and toddlers emerged. Vast amounts of information are available regarding specific patterns of infant development in visual, auditory, cognitive, learning, socio-communicative, motor, sensory, and language performance. As a result of the interest directed toward understanding normal infant development, the infant or toddler is viewed as a remarkably alert and active individual.

Many areas of sensory function are involved in the processing of complex environmental stimuli, thus making the infant or toddler an active observer and, as time progresses, an active participant in the world (Rossetti, 1986). The student of infant development quickly becomes aware developmental principles and generalizations can cross developmental domains. These generalizations include the notion that skill acquisition is independent, and development across all modalities is influenced to some degree by delays in any single area of maturation. Owens (1984) lists five developmental principles that emerge as one studies the domains of infant and toddler development listed previously:

1. Development is predictable.
2. Developmental milestones are attained at about the same time in most children.
3. Developmental opportunity is needed.
4. Children go through developmental changes or periods.
5. Individuals differ greatly.

It is on principles such as those stated by Owens that much of the theoretic bases regarding infant and toddler assessment are predicated. How can one know what constitutes atypical infant or toddler development if one does not know what constitutes normal development? It is precisely information of this nature, gained over time by researchers from many countries, on which judgments regarding developmental adequacy are predicated. Information of this nature formed the basis for much of the attention directed in the late 1960s and early 1970s toward infants and toddlers who were not displaying normal patterns of developmental skill acquisition. Early efforts to promote developmental progress for infants and toddlers not displaying normal patterns of development were a natural result.

STUDY OF THE EFFICACY OF EARLY INTERVENTION

An additional factor that has had a profound effect in altering the current state of activity on infant and toddler assessment and early intervention revolves around numerous research endeavors that have pointed to the effectiveness of early intervention. Several extensive literature reviews have been conducted to determine if early intervention is effective. Although an exhaustive review of the literature is not possible here, an overview of investigations that have pointed to the effectiveness of early intervention will be mentioned. These investigations are reviewed within the context of indicating how information of this nature has contributed positively to the present state of service delivery to infants and toddlers.

Variables in Efficacy Research

A monograph written by Bronfenbrenner (1974) addressed the issue of the effectiveness of early intervention. This article set the stage, at least in part, for controlled studies designed to assess the short- and long-term benefits of early identification and intervention for handicapped preschool-age children. Since that time a variety of researchers, representing various disciplines, have conducted careful studies addressing the same issue. One of the problems encountered in attempting to determine the effectiveness of early intervention is how to control all the potential variables that might influence changes seen in children enrolled in early intervention programs. These variables include (1) family status and involvement in services provided, (2) the factors that identified a child as needing early intervention, (3) the program model employed, (4) the age at which services were initiated, (5) the effectiveness of the curriculum or model used in a given program, (6) the setting in which the intervention was provided, (7) the quality of the staff providing the services, and (8) medical and psychological factors that might hinder a child's progress.

Problems in Efficacy Research

A literature review designed to assess the effectiveness of early intervention programs was performed by Simeonsson, Cooper, and Scheiner (1982).

These authors reviewed 27 studies that described early intervention for biologically impaired infants and toddlers. Although each of the studies reviewed provided some type of documentation of outcome, many of the studies did not collect data in a manner that made objective statistical analysis possible. This was due in part to the difficulty involved in attempting to control the variables previously mentioned. Statistical procedures were used in 59 percent of the studies, and statistical support for the effectiveness of early intervention was reported in 48 percent of the studies reviewed. Effectiveness on the basis of subjective, clinical conclusions was reported in 93 percent of the studies. The authors concluded that despite any limitations on meeting scientific criteria in the studies reviewed, the research does provide qualified support for the effectiveness of early intervention.

Variability of criteria for progress and the methodologic difficulties mentioned make the determination of effectiveness problematic. Meisels (1985) suggests that although efficacy research has been taking place in one form or another for 20 years, the question of whether early intervention is effective remains. This is partially because several assumptions have not been fully considered in the collection of efficacy data. Meisels believes that the question of efficacy persists because too many observers of early intervention, as well as too many investigators, have not asked critical questions about the theoretical rationale of intervention programs, strategies employed, measurement techniques, and child participation criteria. He goes on to state that "another reason the efficacy question continues to be raised is that the primary target of intervention is overlooked." I agree, and I support the view that the primary intervention target should not be the child but the child in the context of the family. The effectiveness of intervention when the family is involved appears to be higher (Simeonsson, Cooper, and Scheiner, 1982).

STUDY OF THE PARENTS'
ROLE IN EARLY INTERVENTION

Initial evaluations of the effectiveness of early intervention programs focused on issues involving a handicapped child's ability to change. More recently attention has been directed toward additional aspects of early intervention efficacy. These include the acquisition of instructional skills by primary caregivers, changes in the quality of interactions between the caregiver and the child, and quality of life changes seen in families of handicapped infants and toddlers.

Barker and Heifetz (1976) and Barker, Heifetz, and Murphy (1980) investigated the effects of training parents as early interventionists. The training focus for parents was to assist them in acquiring techniques geared toward behavior modification. All the mothers who received training demonstrated a significant improvement in their ability to incorporate newly learned skills in providing primary care for their handicapped children. The children of the trained parents improved significantly in acquiring skills over control children. This further supports the supposition that change in a child is related to the parents' ability to incorporate instructional techniques in the home. Additional studies have further demonstrated that early intervention, when parents are included, has an efficacious effect on child development because parents are able to benefit from training in specific aspects of child care and development (Filler and Kasari, 1981; Petrie, Kratochwell, Bergnan, and Nicholson, 1981).

Several investigations have attempted to alter the mother-infant relationship, thus positively influencing interactional activity between the mother and her infant or toddler. Populations studied have included low-income families, poverty-level rural black families, mothers of children with cerebral palsy, and parents of moderately retarded preschool children (Madden, Levenstein, and Levenstein, 1976; Ramey, MacPhee, and Yeates, 1983; Gordon and Kogan, 1975; Christopherson and Sykes, 1979). These investigations have shown that it is beneficial to instruct parents to enhance the family's (primarily the mother's) interactional skills with handicapped infants and toddlers. These results, in tandem with previously known information concerning the importance of early interaction between healthy infants and toddlers and primary caregivers, amplify the need to pay special attention to the quality of interaction between handicapped infants and toddlers and primary caregivers.

Quality of life changes, relative to the efficacy of early intervention, have also been an area of interest to researchers. One investigation (Rescorla and Zigler, 1981) targeted 18 children from birth to 3 years of age, from low-income families. Parents received home visits on a twice-per-month schedule for 12 months and once per month thereafter. The focus of the visits was the parents' social and economic needs. The progress of the children was assessed at periodic intervals for both the control and experimental groups. Analysis at 5-year follow-up study indicated a significant difference favoring the experimental group in areas such as socioeconomic status, number of children (fewer), employment, and general quality of life. The children in the experimental group also exhibited significantly higher scores on tests of vocabulary. Favorable attitudinal changes in parents, affecting overall quality of life, were also reported by Field (1981) and by Spiker (1982).

Bricker (1986), in commenting on the efficacy of programs focused on parents, makes the following summary statements:

1. Comparatively little empirical work determining program impact has been reported.
2. The major thrust of the reported work has been on teaching parents behavioral management skills. The results clearly indicate that parents can acquire specific management and teaching skills. How-

ever, what is less clear is the parents' ability to generalize these skills in functional ways.

3. The impact of programs on a number of important variables concerning quality of life has been studied infrequently, and more research in this area is needed (p. 89).

An additional issue related to the efficacy of early intervention concerns the cost-effectiveness of providing services to infants and toddlers who need special intervention. Although programs of this nature are costly, are savings realized in the long term as children overcome, or at least lessen, the impact of developmental disability? The economic impact from early intervention is of considerable interest to many persons, particularly if a corresponding decrease in future educational expenditures is realized due to early intervention. The fact that the cost of special education exceeds that of regular education is well established. Bricker, Bailey, and Bruder (1984) report that the average annual cost per child for regular education ranges from $1,148 to $2,060. Thus, the average cost per child for regular education for a child to age 18 is between $13,776 and $16,072. In contrast, the average cost for special education to age 18, when intervention starts at birth, age 2, and age 6, is $32,273, $37,600, and $48,816, respectively (Bricker, Bailey, and Bruder, 1984, p. 408). The cost of special education varies according to the type and severity of the handicapping condition and the type of services offered (Rosemiller, Hale, and Frohreich, 1970). The cost of special education also varies as the age at which services are initiated is delayed. In one study, 940 children with a range of handicaps from mild to severe were followed to ascertain cost of services. The median cost of special education (per child per year) was reported to be $2,021 for infants, $2,310 for preschoolers, and $4,445 for elementary and secondary students. These figures represent the median cost of services for 1 year at the ages described (Interact, 1981).

In some cases early intervention services enable children to attend regular education classes. Horton (1976) reports on an early intervention program for hearing-impaired children birth through 6 years of age. The average annual cost for hearing-impaired children to attend regular classes was $847 per child as compared with the average annual cost of $1,017 per child for hearing-impaired children to attend special education classes. The cost to operate an early intervention program is far less than the cost of residential or institutional care. Liberman, Barns, Ho, Cuellar, and Little (1979) reported that the annual cost of providing preschool services for 97 handicapped preschool children was $3,908 per child. The authors speculate that many of these children would have qualified at a later date for residential services if early intervention services had not been provided. The average annual cost for residential school services, as reported by the authors, was $12,888 per person. The cost for institutional care is also substantially greater than the cost for special education services in the school setting.

Other community and economic benefits have been reported when children are placed in the regular classroom. Weber, Foster, and Weikart (1978) suggest that the benefits of early intervention significantly outweigh the initial investment. These investigators indicate that the total economic benefit for 2 years of preschool was $14,819 per child. This represents a 248 percent return on the initial investment of $5,984 per child. The economic benefit figure was derived from decreased educational costs, increased lifetime earnings, and the value of the parents' release time while the children were in the preschool program. In a recent review, the cost of special education services for school-age children with special needs was found to be twice as high as for regular education. Private and public schools spend an average of $6,355 on each special education child compared with $2,780 spent on other students. Moreover, special education costs rose 10 percent between 1977 and 1985, while regular education costs rose only 4 percent during that period. Spending levels varied greatly depending on whether the student was placed in "self-contained" programs that provide more than 15 hours per week of special services ($7,140) or "resource" programs of fewer than 15 hours per week ($647). Placing a handicapped preschool-age child in a residential program costs more than $29,000 per year (ASHA, 1989).

In summary, multiple literature reviews have, for the most part, concluded that early services for children from birth through preschool years, particularly those services actively involving parents, are an effective way to facilitate child development and remediate the effects of early environmental risks (Hanson, 1984; Lazar and Darlington, 1982; McCluskey and Arco, 1979). Table 1–1 summarizes several findings regarding the effectiveness of early intervention. Specific risk populations have been studied to determine the effectiveness of early intervention. Children with Down syndrome, children who are physically and neurologically or sensory impaired, and children with multiple and severe handicaps have all been shown to benefit from early detection and intervention.

FEDERAL LEGISLATION

Over the years numerous federal legislative initiatives have enhanced the status of handicapped and at-risk infants and toddlers. A complete review of the history of federal laws governing service provision to handicapped children is not within the scope of this chapter. However, several federal mandates that have had direct impact on handicapped children will be mentioned. Two specific pieces of legislation that have had profound impact on service delivery for handicapped children will be discussed. Table 1–2 presents an overview of important federal legislation that has affected service delivery for infants and toddlers.

**TABLE 1-1. Summary statements regarding
the effectiveness of early intervention**

1. Programs for young children at environmental risk produced long-lasting positive effects on child-school competence and abilities, children's attitudes, and family attitudes.

2. The infant born at risk for biologic damage may benefit from early physical and educational therapies.

3. Early intervention services provided to infants born with established risks and their families have been shown to be effective at remediating the effects of the disability and at accelerating the child's development.

4. Family members are affected by the birth of a disabled or at-risk infant and often seek out and benefit from early intervention services.

5. Early intervention services produce a variety of effects on the child, family, and community.

6. Initial studies of early intervention's cost-effectiveness suggest that significant savings may be derived from the provision of these services.

7. The following components are present in those intervention services that produce the greatest change in children:
   A. Active parent involvement
   B. Systematic early educational services
   C. Developmentally based curricula
   D. Individualized goal setting
   E. Frequent updating of child programs
   F. Intervention beginning at as early an age as possible
   G. Follow-up study when children leave the program

Source: Adapted from M. Hanson (1984). The effects of early intervention. In M. Hanson (Ed.), *Atypical infant development*. Austin, TX: PRO-ED.

Perhaps the two most significant pieces of federal legislation to affect service provision to handicapped children are P.L. 94-142, the Education for All Handicapped Children Act, passed in 1975, and P.L. 99-457, the Education of the Handicapped Amendments of 1986. Each of these federal mandates promotes and expands the federal role in identifying and providing appropriate educational services to handicapped children. The effect of these two acts is to afford all handicapped children the right to educational intervention from an early age. Each of these acts will be discussed in greater detail.

P.L. 94-142: THE EDUCATION OF ALL HANDICAPPED CHILDREN ACT

P.L. 94-142 has been called one of the most important pieces of federal legislation enacted for the handicapped child. Its major intent was to pro-

TABLE 1-2. Federal initiatives affecting handicapped children

Year	Legislation	Intent/impact
1957	P.L. 85-926	Trained teachers to work with mentally retarded persons
1958	P.L. 85-864	Developed educational media for mentally retarded persons
1964	P.L. 88-164	Established university-affiliated programs for teaching and research on mental retardation and developmental disabilities
1965	P.L. 89-10	Established federal aid to education as a national policy
1965	P.L. 89-313	Authorized federal assistance to state-supported schools and institutions
1965	P.L. 89-750	Provided the basis for federal involvement in special education
1967	P.L. 90-248	Prompted early detection and prevention of developmental problems
1968	P.L. 90-538	First federal legislation aimed at young handicapped children
1972	P.L. 90-924	Required Head Start programs to serve handicapped children
1973	P.L. 93-112	Prevented discrimination based on a disability
1974	P.L. 93-644	Redefined the term *handicapped* to include more severely impaired children

vide a free, appropriate education in the least restrictive environment for every school-aged handicapped child. With the enactment of this mandate, education for handicapped children became the right of every child and not just the privilege of the few. The law also affords parents the right of due process and full involvement in decisions that relate to classification and educational placement for their child. In essence, parents are able to hold public school professionals accountable for the placement their child receives. The law includes provisions to ensure the following (Gallagher, 1984):

The right to education — all handicapped children are to be provided with free and appropriate public education
The right to nondiscriminatory evaluation
The right to an individualized education plan (IEP) with a clear statement of objectives for each child along with documentation of the child's current and expected performance
The right to education in the least restrictive environment

The right to due process
The right of parental participation

The law further emphasizes educating handicapped children with non-handicapped children as much as possible. It also requires that school districts provide a continuum of alternative placements, including consultants, resource rooms, itinerant programs, self-contained classes, special schools, residential programs, and home and hospital services (McCarthy, 1980). The law is designed to match as closely as possible the child's specific educational needs with available resources.

Perhaps one of the strongest aspects of the law concerns provisions designed to increase the accountability of intervention strategies. This is accomplished through the use of an IEP. The IEP, which is prepared for each child yearly, must do the following (Rossetti, 1986, p. 143):

Describe the child's present level of performance
Outline long-range goals in areas such as language, gross and fine motor functioning, cognitive development, preacademic skills, self-help skills, and social and emotional development
State short-term instructional objectives
Describe the specific special education and related services to be provided, along with projected dates for initiation of services and their anticipated duration
State appropriate objective criteria, evaluation procedures, and a schedule for determining if the instructional objectives are being achieved

The law does not mandate the provision of educational programs for non–school-age children, although individual states may decide to include programming for preschool-age handicapped children. One section of P.L. 94-142 offered small incentive grants to encourage states to develop programs for handicapped children 3 to 5 years of age. Several states (Iowa, Nebraska, Michigan, and New Jersey) have used these funds and additional funds generated by the state to initiate programs for children 3 to 5 years of age as well as programs for children 0 to 3 years of age.

O'Connell (1983) conducted a national survey designed to assess the status of services and personnel for handicapped preschoolers. Information from all 50 states and the District of Columbia was obtained. States were asked to indicate whether a legislative mandate (state level) existed to serve two subgroups of the handicapped population: children from birth to 3 years and from 3 to 5 years of age. Sixteen percent of the states reported that state requirements mandated the provision of educational services to all handicapped children from birth to 5 years. Within the birth to 3-year-old range, an additional 8 percent of the states had mandated educational services for limited subgroups of the target population. Another 24 percent of the states had mandated that all handicapped children within the 3-to-5-year-old subgroup be provided educational services. In 14 percent of the states, limited subgroups of the population were served. Thirty-five percent of the states had state standards and regulations for certifying teachers of preschool handicapped children, and 24 percent of the states indicated that the process of developing such standards was underway. Forty-one percent of the states reported no such standards governing teachers of young handicapped children. These results indicate some progress on the state level in providing service to handicapped infants and toddlers.

The *Seventh Annual Report to Congress on the Implementation of the Education of the Handicapped Act* (Jones, 1985) included information on age requirements by state for handicapped children to receive special services. This information, which includes age of initiation of service and upper-age limit, is presented in Tables 1-3 and 1-4.

TABLE 1-3. Mandates for serving handicapped children aged 6 years and younger by state

0-5	2-5	3-5	4-5	5	6
IA	VA	AK	DE	AL	AR
MD		CA	MN	CO	AZ
MI		CT	OK	FL	IN
NE		DC	TN	GA	MS
NJ		HI	WA	ID	MT
SD		IL		KS	ND
		LA		KY	OR
		MA		ME	PA
		NH		MO	VT
		RI		NC	
		TX		NM	
		WI		NV	
				NY	
				OH	
				SC	
				UT	
				WV	
				WY	

Source: Adapted from G. Jones (1985). Seventh annual report to Congress on the implementation of the Education of the Handicapped Act. Washington, DC: Division of Education Services Special Education Programs, U.S. Department of Education.

TABLE 1-4. State mandates: Upper age
limit for service eligibility

18	19	20	21		23	25	Other
GA	HI	AL	AK	OH	WV	MI	FL
IN		AR	AZ	PA			
MT		CO	CA	RI			
NC		DE	CT	DC			
NV		ID	SC	IL			
OK		IA	SD	KS			
		ME	TN	KY			
		MD	TX	LA			
		MN	UT	MA			
		MO	VT	NJ			
		MS	VA	NM			
		NE	WA	ND			
		NH	WI				
		NY					
		OR					
		WY					

Source: Adapted from G. Jones (1985). Seventh annual report to
Congress on the implementation of the Education of the Handi-
capped Act. Washington, DC: Division of Education Services Special
Education Programs, U.S. Department of Education.

P.L. 99-457: EDUCATION OF THE HANDICAPPED AMENDMENTS OF 1986

The most important piece of federal legislation affecting special education
since the passage of P.L. 94-142 in 1975 was signed into law in October
1986. This act is known as P.L. 99-457, the Education of the Handicapped
Amendments of 1986. A detailed discussion of this legislation will follow.

This legislation has had an enormous impact on service delivery for handicapped infants and toddlers. It "is the most important thing that Congress
will do for handicapped infants and young children up to the age of five in
this decade and perhaps for the remainder of this century. This legislation
will require commitment, effort, expertise, long hours, and, yes, money
(Williams, *Liaison Bulletin,* 1986)." Weicker (*Liaison Bulletin,* 1986) indicated that "this legislation represents an important step forward in fulfilling
a Federal commitment to those most vulnerable in our society, who require
special care. It is the right thing to do, in both human and economic terms."

These comments, shared by legislators who were instrumental in the passage of P.L. 99-457, point out the substantial impact that this legislation has had on handicapped infants and toddlers. There are three main titles in P.L. 99-457. A title-by-title summary follows.

Title I: Handicapped Infants and Toddlers

Title I established a new discretionary program designed to address the needs of handicapped infants and toddlers and their families. The authors of the legislation felt that an urgent need existed to (1) enhance the development of handicapped infants and toddlers and to minimize their potential for developmental delay; (2) to reduce the costs of such delay to society, including schools; (3) to minimize the likelihood of institutionalization; and (4) to enhance families' ability to meet their handicapped children's needs. The law provides states financial assistance to develop and implement a statewide, comprehensive, coordinated, interdisciplinary program of early intervention services for handicapped infants and toddlers and their families; facilitates coordination of payments for early intervention services from various public and private sources; and enhances the capacity to provide quality early intervention services and expand and improve existing services.

Handicapped infants and toddlers are defined as individuals from birth through age 2 who require early intervention services because they:

Are experiencing developmental delays as measured by appropriate diagnostic instruments and procedures in one or more of the following areas: cognitive development, physical development, language and speech development, psychosocial development, or self-help skills.

Have a diagnosed physical or mental condition that has a high probability of resulting in developmental delay. The term may also include, at a state's discretion, individuals (birth–2 years) who are "at risk" of having substantial developmental delays if early intervention services are not provided. The term *developmental delay* is defined by each state.

In addition to providing guidelines for determining which children will be served by P.L. 99-457, the legislation further defined what is meant by early intervention services. As stated in the legislation, the term *early intervention* means developmental services that:

Are provided under public supervision

Are provided at no cost, except where federal or state law requires a system of payments by families, including a schedule of sliding fees

Are designed to meet a handicapped infant's or toddler's developmental needs (physical development, cognitive development, and self-help skills)

Meet state standards

Are provided by qualified personnel, including special educators, speech-language pathologists and audiologists, occupational therapists, physical therapists, social workers, nurses, and nutritionists

Are provided in conformity with an individualized family service plan (IFSP)

Include family training, counseling, and home visits; special instruction; speech pathology and audiology; occupational therapy; physical therapy; psychological services; case management services; medical services for diagnostic or evaluation purposes; early identification, screening, and assessment services; and health services necessary to enable the infant or toddler to benefit from the other early intervention services

Perhaps one of the most beneficial aspects of the legislation deals with the implementation of case management services. Although early intervention has been available in some parts of the country, in many instances this intervention service was fragmented. This was because infants and toddlers received services from many professionals, but no mechanism existed to afford proper management of the total services the child received. Case management services, as outlined in the legislation, include services provided to families to assist them in gaining access to early intervention services and other services identified in the IFSP. The main difference between the IFSP and the IEP is that the IFSP requires and authorizes that intervention services be directed at the identified needs of the family and parents as well as at the child's specific needs. It is intended that case management be an active, ongoing process of continually seeking the appropriate services or situations that benefit the development of each infant or toddler, for the duration of the child's eligibility. Case management includes ensuring timely delivery of intervention and coordinating these services with other areas of intervention that the infant or toddler needs or that are being provided.

Title II: Handicapped Children Aged 3 Through 5

By 1992, under Title II of the legislation, states are required to provide a free and appropriate public education and related services to disabled children from age 3. This section will replace P.L. 94-142, the Education for All Handicapped Children Act, the preschool incentive grant program (which was permissive in allowing states to serve children from age 3) with a national mandate that requires all handicapped children to be served from age 3.

The law further indicates that each state must have in effect a comprehensive, coordinated, multidisciplinary system of delivering early intervention services for all handicapped infants and toddlers and their families. The component parts of the statewide plan, which each state must have in place before it can receive funding, include the following:

Definition of the term *developmentally delayed* to be used by the state in carrying out the program

Reasonable goals and timetables for making appropriate early intervention services available to all handicapped infants and toddlers

Performance of a timely, comprehensive, and multidisciplinary evaluation of the functioning of each handicapped infant and toddler and the needs of the family to assist appropriately in the development of the handicapped infant or toddler

Development of IFSPs and the provision of case management services

A comprehensive child-locating system and a system for referrals to service providers that includes timelines and provides for participation of primary referral services (hospitals, physicians, public health facilities, and so on)

A public awareness strategy program on early identification of handicapped infants and toddlers

A central directory that includes early intervention services, resources, and experts available in the state, plus research and demonstration projects in the state

A comprehensive system of personnel development that includes training of public and private service providers, primary referral sources, and persons who will provide services after receiving such training

A single line of authority in an agency designated by the governor to carry out (1) the general administration, supervision, and monitoring of programs and activities; (2) the identification and coordination of all available resources within the state from federal, state, local, and private sources; (3) the resolution of interagency disputes and procedures for ensuring the provision of services pending the resolution of such disputes; and (4) the entering into of formal state interagency agreements that define each state agency's financial responsibility for paying for early intervention services (consistent with state law)

A policy pertaining to the contracting or making of other arrangements with local service providers

Procedural safeguards for early intervention programs

A system for compiling data regarding the early intervention programs (which may be based on a sampling of data)

Title II also includes provisions for the IFSP. This represents an enhanced awareness of the importance of the family in remediating developmental delay in infants and toddlers. Title II of the legislation specifies that services be expanded to include the family. In effect, the IFSP expands services beyond the child and includes primary caregivers as important members of the treatment team. Included in the provisions outlining the IFSP are guidelines that provide that each handicapped infant or toddler and the infant or toddler's family receive a multidisciplinary assessment designed to identify the unique needs and services needed. The IFSP must be reviewed once every year, and the family must be provided with:

A statement of the family's strengths and needs related to development of the family's handicapped infant or toddler

A statement of the major outcomes expected for the infant or toddler and the family; to the extent appropriate, the criteria, procedures and timelines used to determine the degree to which progress toward achieving the outcomes is being made; and a statement of whether modifications or revisions of the outcomes or services are necessary

A statement of specific early intervention services necessary to meet the unique needs of the infant or toddler and family, including the frequency, intensity, and method of delivering services

The projected dates for initiating available services and the anticipated duration of such services

The name of the case manager from the profession most immediately relevant to the infant or toddler or family who will be responsible for implementing the plan and coordinating with other agencies or persons

The steps to be taken supporting the transition of the handicapped infant or toddler to services provided under other parts of the act

Title III: Discretionary Programs

Title III of P.L. 99-457 added a number of discretionary programs designed to support the full intent of the law. These programs:

Define how funds may be used to establish regional resource centers within each state

Define and expand services to deaf-blind children and youth

Provide amendments to provisions previously established for the early education of handicapped children

Provide funds for personnel training, including money to state education agencies and institutions of higher education to establish and mantain preservice and inservice continuing education activities

Provide grants to improve recruitment of educational personnel and dissemination of information concerning educational opportunities for the handicapped

Expand research and demonstration projects for education of handicapped children

Further define the provisions designed to establish panels of experts who are responsible for evaluating proposals for funding under various parts of the act

Expand services designed to provide educational media for handicapped persons

Provide funds designed to advance the use of new technology, media, and materials in the education of handicapped students and in the provision of early intervention to handicapped infants and toddlers

Title IV: Miscellaneous

Under Title IV of P.L. 99-457, various miscellaneous areas are discussed, clarified, and expanded. Two of the provisions under Title IV are of particular interest to practitioners involved in assessing infants and toddlers. These include provisions dealing with the personnel involved in service provision to infants and toddlers and the issue of evaluation and classification of handicapped children receiving services within each state.

In the section dealing with the use of qualified personnel, two major guidelines are established. These relate to the establishment and maintenance of standards to ensure that personnel necessary to carry out the intent of the entire act are appropriately and adequately prepared and trained. These provisions regarding qualified personnel address two major areas.

First, the act provides for the establishment and maintenance of standards consistent with any state-approved or -recognized certification, licensing, registration, or other comparable requirements that apply to the area in which the individual is providing special education and related services. Second, if the existing standards are not based on the highest requirements in the state for a specific profession or discipline, the state must take steps to require the retraining or hiring of personnel who meet appropriate professional requirements.

The cumulative effect of these two landmark pieces of legislation on the federal level, P.L. 94-142 and P.L. 99-457, has been to enhance significantly the status of service provision to handicapped infants and toddlers and their families. The full impact of these mandates is not fully known. The increased numbers of children to be served, the long-term outcome of services to these handicapped infants and toddlers, the effects on families, the fiscal obligations of providing services to infants and toddlers, and a host of additional issues are unknown at present. Even in light of a lack of data and information regarding some of these issues, the current status of high-risk and handicapped infants and toddlers has been enormously enhanced as a result of the federal initiative to ensure quality early intervention.

SUMMARY

Why is there an enhanced interest in the early detection of developmental deviancy? As has been pointed out in this chapter, multiple factors have actively shaped the current status of early assessment and intervention for handicapped infants and toddlers. Not the least of these is the federal mandate to do so. Hence, practitioners no longer have the option of gaining expertise in infant and toddler assessment. We are forced to do so. What was previously the domain of a minority of practitioners will in the future become the common experience of all.

The objective of early identification and intervention for handicapped infants and toddlers is to help overcome the child's delay in developmental skill acquisition through a family model of intervention. This involves assisting the parents to better understand the child's disability, to help them accept the responsibility for full involvement in intervention activity, and to face the challenges inherent in the disability in a positive way.

According to Sheehan and Gallagher (1982), various program goals for early identification and intervention exist for both infants and parents. These include:

1. Maintaining normal developmental functioning in all areas of development
2. Preventing an increase in developmental delay in one or more areas
3. Demonstrating progress in one or more developmental areas
4. Reducing stress and anxiety associated with parenting a handicapped infant or toddler
5. Increasing verbal interaction between the family and the handicapped infant or toddler
6. Increasing the amount of responsibility that a parent takes for educating the handicapped child

The realization of these objectives is enhanced through the early detection of developmental delay in those children with or without known risk of manifesting developmental deviancy. Early identification and intervention are one and the same. One without the other is not a viable option for the early interventionist. Soboloff (1981) has stated that "it can no longer be accepted that treatment for these children does not begin until

three years of age. From our own experience, we feel that early stimulation
benefits not only the child, but also the parents and the entire family" (p.
265). This process begins with the early detection and assessment of developmental deviancy.

STUDY QUESTIONS

1. How did the Civil Rights movement of the 1950s influence legislation dealing with handicapped persons?
2. How has research dealing with normal infant development, the
   efficacy of early intervention, and parental involvement in intervention enhanced the status of handicapped infants and toddlers?
3. Describe the four main titles of P.L. 99-457.
4. What are the responsibilities of the lead agency in implementing
   P.L. 99-457?
5. What is the main difference between the IEP required under P.L.
   94-142 and the IFSP required under P.L. 99-457?

REFERENCES

Allen, K. (1984). Federal legislation and young handicapped children. *Topics in
   Early Childhood Special Education, 4,* 9.
ASHA. (1989). Special education costs double the dollars. *ASHA, 31,* 11.
Baker, B., & Heifetz, L. (1976). The read project: Teaching manuals for parents of
   retarded children. In T. Tjossem (Ed.), *Intervention strategies for high risk and
   young children.* Baltimore: University Park Press.
Barker, B., Heifetz, L., & Murphy, D. (1980). Behavioral training for parents of mentally retarded children: One year follow-up. *American Journal of Mental Deficiency, 85,* 31.
Bricker, D. (1986). *Early education of at-risk and handicapped infants, toddlers, and
   preschool children.* Glenview, IL: Scott, Foresman.
Bricker, D., Bailey, E., & Bruder, M. (1984). The efficacy of early intervention and
   the handicapped infant: A wise or wasted resource. *Advances in Developmental
   and Behavioral Pediatrics, 5,* 373.
Bronfenbrenner, U. (1974). *Is early intervention effective?* Washington, DC: Office
   of Human Development.
Christopherson, E., & Sykes, B. (1979). An intensive, home based family training
   program for developmentally delayed children. In L. Hamerlynck (Ed.), *Behavioral systems for the developmentally disabled: Vol. I. School and family environments.* New York: Brunner/Mazel.
Field, T. (1981). Intervention for high risk infants and their parents. *Educational
   Evaluation and Policy Analysis, 3,* 69.
Filler, J. W. (1983). Service models for handicapped infants. In G. Garwood & R.
   Fewell (Eds.), *Educating handicapped infants.* Rockville, MD: Aspen Publications.

Filler, J., & Kasari, C. (1981). Acquisition, maintenance and generalization of parent-taught skills with two severely handicapped infants. *The Journal of the Association for the Severely Handicapped, 6,* 30.

Gallagher, J. (1984). Policy analysis and program implementation/P.L. 94-142. *Topics in Early Childhood Special Education, 4,* 43.

Gordon, N., & Kogan, K. (1975). A mother instruction program: Behavior changes with and without therapeutic intervention. *Child Psychiatry and Human Development, 6,* 89.

Hanson, M. (1984). The effects of early intervention. In M. Hanson (Ed.), *Atypical infant development.* Baltimore: University Park Press.

Horton, K. (1976). Early intervention for hearing impaired infants and young children. In T. Tjossem (Ed.), *Intervention strategies for high risk infants and young children.* Austin, TX: PRO-ED.

Interact. (1981). Early intervention for children with special needs and their families. Manuscript prepared by Interact: The national committee for service to very young children with special needs and their families. Monmouth, OR: Westar.

Jones, G. (1985). Seventh annual report to Congress on the implementation of the Education of the Handicapped Act. Washington, DC: Division of Educational Services Special Education Programs, U.S. Department of Education.

Lazar, I., & Darlington, R. (1982). Lasting effects of early education: A report from the consortium for longitudinal studies. *Monographs of the Society for Research in Child Development, 47,* 2.

Liberman, A., Barnes, M., Ho, E., Cuellar, I., & Little, T. (1979). The economic impact of child development services on families of retarded children. *Mental Retardation, 17,* 158.

Madden, J., Levenstein, P., & Levenstein, S. (1976). Longitudinal IQ outcomes of the mother-child home program. *Child Development, 47,* 1015.

McCarthy, J. (1980). Early intervention and school programs for preschool handicapped children. In E. Sell (Ed.), *Follow-up of the high risk newborn: A practical approach.* Springfield, IL: Charles C Thomas.

McCluskey, K., & Arco, C. (1979). Stimulation and infant development. In J. Howells (Ed.), *Modern perspectives in the psychiatry of infancy.* New York: Brunner/Mazel.

Meisels, S. (1985). The efficacy of early intervention: Why are we still asking the question? *Topics in Early Childhood Special Education, 5,* 1.

O'Connell, J. (1983). Education of handicapped preschoolers: A national survey of services and personnel requirements. *Exceptional Children, 49,* 538.

Owens, R. (1984). *Language development: An introduction.* Columbus, OH: Charles E. Merrill.

Petrie, P., Kratochwell, T., Bergnan, J., & Nicholson, G. (1981). Teaching parents to teach their children: Applications in the pediatric setting. *Journal of Pediatric Psychology, 6,* 275.

Ramey, C., MacPhee, D., & Yeates, K. (1983). Preventing developmental retardation: A general systems model. In L. Bond & J. Joffe (Eds.), *Facilitating infant and early childhood development.* Hanover, NH: University Press of New England.

Rescorla, I., & Zigler, E. (1981). The Yale child welfare research program: Implications for social policy. *Education Evaluation and Policy Analysis, 3,* 5.

Rossetti, L. (1986). *High risk infants: Identification, assessment, and intervention.* Austin, TX: PRO-ED.

Rossmiller, R., Hale, J., & Frohreich, L. (1970). Educational programs for exceptional children: Resource configurations and cost. National Education Finance

Project (Special Study No. 102). Wisconsin: Department of Educational Administration.

Sheehan, R., & Gallagher, R. (1982). Conducting evaluations of infant intervention programs. In S. Garwood & R. Fewell (Eds.), *Educating handicapped infants.* Rockville, MD: Aspen Systems.

Simeonsson, R., Cooper, D., & Scheiner, A. (1982). A review of the effectiveness of early intervention programs. *Pediatrics, 69,* 635.

Soboloff, H. (1981). Early intervention — fact or fiction. *Developmental Medicine and Child Neurology, 23,* 261.

Spiker, D. (1982). Parent involvement in early intervention activities with their young children with Down Syndrome. *Education and Training of the Mentally Retarded, 17,* 24.

Staff. (1986, Oct. 22). P.L. 99-457 promises major federal partnership in early childhood education. *Liaison Bulletin,* 1.

Weber, C., Foster, P., & Weikart, D. (1978). An economic analysis of the Ypsilanti Perry Preschool Project. Monograph of the High/Scope Educational Research Foundation, No. 5.

Weicker, L. (1986). P.L. 99:457 promises a major federal partnership in early childhood education. *Liaison Bulletin, 1.*

Williams, R. (1986). P.L. 99:457 promises major federal partnership in early childhood education. *Liaison Bulletin, 1.*

CHAPTER 2

Recipients of Infant-Toddler Assessment

Causation in
Developmental Disorders
   Approaches: Retrospective and
      Prospective
   Models

Conditions and Causes
Contributing to
Developmental Disorders
   Chromosomal and Genetic
      Abnormalities
   Prenatal and Perinatal Factors
   Postnatal Environmental
      Factors

Summary

Study Questions

References

One of the first tasks facing the practitioner involved in infant and toddler assessment is determining which children need neurodevelopmental evaluation. One might say this is an easy task, since those children who fit various biologic categories are known to display patterns of developmental deviancy. These children are suspected of developmental delay at an early age and hence are put into the service delivery system at a relatively early age.

Who are these children, and what factors place them at risk for delayed development? How does the practitioner become aware of who needs developmental assessment? What etiologic categories exist for viewing causation of developmental delay? Are there effective ways of viewing causation to assist the practitioner in interpreting assessment results as well as in making management decisions? The practitioner must be prepared to answer these questions. This chapter is designed to address these issues.

CAUSATION IN DEVELOPMENTAL DISORDERS

APPROACHES: RETROSPECTIVE AND PROSPECTIVE

When a child displays a delayed pattern of development, it is quite natural for parents and professionals alike to wonder why. The practitioner immediately looks for factors that have caused, or at least have heavily contributed to, the delayed pattern of development noted. It seems reasonable to assume that if one can understand why a disorder is present, then the practitioner is one step closer to a better understanding of the special needs a child may have.

In attempting to better understand the factors that cause developmental delay, two main experimental designs have been employed (Sameroff and Chandler, 1975). One approach is known as the retrospective approach. In studies of this nature, children who demonstrate various developmental pathologies are identified. Once a child is identified, the researcher carefully examines the child's early history in an attempt to discover factors that are causally related to the developmental disorder present. These studies are retrospective in that they look back in time. Thus, the researcher notes that the child has a developmental disorder and looks for factors that may have caused it. Through such studies, four general categories of factors have been identified that are known to contribute to developmental delay: anoxia, prematurity, complications of delivery, and socioeconomic factors. The presence of one or more of these factors is said to put a child at increased risk of suffering a developmental disorder of some sort.

A second approach to the study of causation is known as the prospective approach. In studies of this nature, infants who display particular risk factors are followed over time to see if they do indeed display later developmental disorders. These studies are more difficult to do because the children must be followed over a long period. A prospective study is, in essence, a predictive one. Prospective studies have for the most part demonstrated that the presence of high-risk factors — those thought to be important in the retrospective studies — may not be as strongly connected to causation. Of the four factors previously mentioned, the most powerful predictor of later developmental status appears to be the child's socioeconomic environment. Thus the environment is known to be of great importance in developmental disorders.

What the above discussion demonstrates is that causation is a difficult issue to understand fully. When the factors identified as high risk in retrospective studies are tested through prospective studies, they lose their potency (Hubbell, 1981). A discussion of various models of causation and how various factors affect their contribution to developmental pathologic states should afford the practitioner a more complete understanding of causation in a broader context.

MODELS

Before discussing specific factors known to cause or at least to contribute heavily to developmental pathology, the practitioner should have an overall philosophy of causation in mind. Sameroff (1975) and Sameroff and Chandler (1975) describe three different views of the process of causation. The practitioner should be familiar with these views. Assessment activity should be undertaken with a proper appreciation of and familiarity with the factors that have contributed to the developmental delay suspected. In other words, assessment activity, as well as management decisions, should be made by a practitioner with a full understanding of how causal factors interact and relate to the child's disability.

Linear Cause-and-Effect Model

The linear cause-and-effect model holds that there is a direct one-to-one relationship between a cause and an effect. In essence, each cause has an effect and each effect has a specific cause. Over time this view has been called the medical model of viewing causation, since this approach underlines a great deal of work in medicine. Inherent in this model is the necessity of determining cause, because intervention and treatment arise, at least in part, from the knowledge of causation.

Viewing developmental pathology from this standpoint is appealing, at least initially. It allows the practitioner to search for factors in the child's history and identify those events known to be highly related to developmental delay. Sameroff (1975) points out that the linear cause-and-effect model makes an important distinction in thinking about causation. This distinction, the relationship between nature and nurture, has been at the center of vigorous debate for quite some time. At the center of this debate is the question of how much of the child's functioning can be explained in terms of genetic endowment and how much in terms of environmental influences. If these two categories of factors (i.e., genetic endowment and environmental influences) are viewed from the linear cause-and-effect model, then there are several possible ways to view the causation of developmental pathology.

Genetic Endowment. One approach is to view such pathology as primarily caused by genetic factors, neurophysiologic makeup, or disease. This can be described as causation that originates from within the child (Hubbell, 1981). Thus, from the linear cause-and-effect model, if risk factors from within the child are identified (e.g., heredity, disease, genetic factors, biologic damage), the child has a high probability of displaying developmental pathology. This prognosis would be true regardless of the nature of the environment in which the child is raised because the child's constitution (nature) is less than optimal.

Environmental Influence. The second approach is to view developmental disabilities as primarily caused by environmental factors. Hence, developmental outcome from the linear cause-and-effect standpoint depends on the quality of the environment regardless of the child's constitution. Just as severe cases of retardation due to genetic causes support a constitutional view of cause and effect, so dramatic cases of environmental deprivation support an environmental view (Hubbell, 1981, p. 108). If causation is viewed from the environmental standpoint, then at least two aspects of the environment must be understood to contribute to the etiology of developmental pathology — the sociocultural and the caretaking environments. A variety of investigators have explored the importance of these two aspects of environment. Their conclusions strongly support the effect of the environment on overall development (Bronfenbrenner, 1975; Skeels, 1966; Whitehurst, Novak, and Zorn, 1972; Bruner, 1978; Greenfield and Smith, 1976; Heath, 1983; Menyuk, 1971).

Nature vs. Nurture: Interdependence. In summary, the linear cause-and-effect model of causation emphasizes either the child's constitution or environment as being the primary etiologic factor in a particular case. Many persons, parents and professionals alike, search for "the cause" when confronted with a child who is not displaying normal patterns of developmental skill mastery. Focusing solely on either the environment or the constitution, without realizing the interdependence of these two factors, limits the assessor in gaining a complete understanding of the nature of the suspected developmental pathology.

Interactional Model

A second and more plausible manner in which to view causation has been termed the interactional model (Sameroff, 1975). In this view the child's development is the result of the interaction between the constitution and the environment. This model is more comprehensive and takes into account the importance of both the environment and the child's constitution. Application of this model would allow for the efficacious nature of the environment in a child with a history of constitutional compromise (e.g., prematurity, low birth weight, anoxia, disease). Werner, Bierman, and French (1971) demonstrated that complications at birth were not necessarily related to later developmental problems unless they were associated with poor environmental conditions. Escalona (1982) followed a group of premature infants and a group of normal birth-weight infants until the children were 3½ years of age. The results of the follow-up evaluations revealed that neither neurologic pathology (except severe brain damage) nor gestational age had a significant effect on intelligence quotient (IQ) scores at 3½ years of age. Further results suggested that environmental deficits and stresses impair early cognitive and psychosocial development for both full-term and premature infants but that the latter group is more vulnerable to environmental insufficiencies than are full-term babies.

What the results of studies of this nature indicate is that the practitioner can no longer search for a single cause of a developmental pathology. Two concerns described by Sameroff (1975) concerning the interactional model of viewing causation should be mentioned at this point. First, it is assumed that neither the child's constitution nor the environment undergoes change. Second, it is assumed that the child and the environment do not affect each other.

Transactional Model

The transactional model of viewing causation was proposed by Sameroff (1975). This view incorporates some of the previous models but differs qualitatively from them. The transactional model includes change over time and emphasizes the reciprocal influences between the child and the environment. At the center of the transactional model is the realization that both the child and the environment change over time. Thus the child's outcome may vary depending on the particular time frame in which outcome is assessed. Both the environment and the child influence each other, so that at different points in time the assessor's view might change. Recall the previous discussion of the two basic paradigms used in studying causation, the retrospective and prospective methods. It is a transactional view of etiology that best explains the apparent contradictions between prospective and retrospective studies. The fact that the child changes the environment and that the environment influences the child is at the heart of a transactional view of etiology.

One problem with the transactional view is that the identification of specific etiologies becomes quite difficult. Even in the presence of clear-cut factors that are known to contribute to developmental delay, such as prematurity and neonatal illness, the exact manner in which these factors influence the child's environment is not fully known. The practitioner must therefore be aware of factors that might contribute to children significantly changing their environments and the manner in which the environment affects the child. These factors are the ones that would place a child in the high-risk category. The child is considered to be at greater risk for the later emergence of developmental pathology not only because of the readily identifiable factor (e.g., prematurity, neonatal illness), but also because of the way in which these apparent factors influence the child's environment (Escalona, 1982).

Note, however, that positive influences may result from the presence of a handicapped infant or toddler in the family, in part due to the positive manner in which the family works together as a unit to meet the handicapped child's special needs. Practitioners report with relative frequency the manner in which many families pull together and develop better communication and stress management skills to meet the special needs of a handicapped infant or toddler. The long-range result of developing improved skills in these areas benefits not only the handicapped child but also the entire family unit. It is not uncommon for parents to report that they learned more from their handicapped child than the child ever learned from them. This is a positive factor of having a handicapped infant or toddler within the family unit.

Summary

The models of viewing causation should alert the assessor to the complexity inherent in attempting to identify a single cause of a developmental disorder observed in a child. Rather than take the easy path — that of ascribing a developmental delay to a readily identifiable factor — the practitioner must be alert to the manner in which a host of factors interact and ultimately result in the developmental pathology seen. The practitioner must also be constantly aware of the present status of the interaction between the child and the environment and of how this transactional pattern affects the child's developmental delay. The infant-toddler assessor is encouraged to adopt a transactional view of causation, and the material in the remainder of this text is presented from a transactional viewpoint.

CONDITIONS AND CAUSES CONTRIBUTING
TO DEVELOPMENTAL DISORDERS

The early interventionist must be extremely familiar with factors that contribute to developmental deviancy and that will likewise affect the child's interaction with the environment. It is precisely these factors that will in large measure determine the recipients of infant and toddler assessment.

Factors known to contribute to the presence of later developmental delay can have their onset in the prenatal, perinatal, or postnatal period. Etiologically significant prenatal factors can include genetic deviations, toxins and harmful drugs, lack of sufficient fetal nutrition, maternal infection, placental problems, and environmental factors such as maternal age, socioeconomic status, and family size. Perinatal problems can include difficulties or trauma during labor and delivery, neonatal medical complications, prematurity, respiratory difficulties including anoxia, and low birth weight and all its accompanying complications. Postnatal problems can include chronic illness, environmental toxins, accidents, central nervous system (CNS) disorders of later onset, poverty, abuse, neglect, and family dysfunction (Ramey, Trohanis, and Hostler, 1982). A discussion of many of these areas follows.

CHROMOSOMAL AND GENETIC ABNORMALITIES

The following discussion is limited to some of the more common conditions related to chromosomal abnormalities. It is not meant to be exhaustive in scope but is intended to acquaint the practitioner with these conditions and their relationship to developmental delay.

Down Syndrome

Down syndrome arises from the presence of an extra chromosome 21 and is technically referred to as trisomy 21. The incidence is variously cited from one in 650 to one in 1,200 live births. It is the most common autosomal abnormality in humans. Approximately 30 to 40 percent of Down syndrome children have accompanying heart disease. Both physical and psychomotor development are delayed, as is language development. The largest percentage of Down children are mentally retarded. In most cases persons with Down syndrome can live in society and function as productive citizens. This largely depends, however, on at what age the disorder is detected and the amount and type of early intervention provided. The quality and involvement of the home situation has also been shown to contribute to later levels of developmental skill mastery achieved by Down syndrome children (Pueshel and Thuline, 1983). Advanced maternal age is the principal risk factor for Down syndrome. Women aged 35 and over have a probability of one in 300 of bearing a Down syndrome child. Other risk factors include a history of spontaneous abortion.

Kleinfelter's Syndrome

Kleinfelter's syndrome is characterized by small genitalia, infertility, and scant facial and pubic hair. Some afflicted persons also have congenital anomalies. Approximately 20 percent of children with Kleinfelter's syndrome are mentally retarded. Approximately one in 1,000 live male infants has this disorder.

Inborn Errors of Metabolism

Inborn errors of metabolism are the result of genetic defects. Many are treatable if detected early. A large number of these disorders can be detected at an early age and appropriate treatment administered. If detected early, developmental disability can be largely prevented or at least mitigated. Two examples of inborn errors of metabolism are phenylketonuria (PKU) and hypothyroidism.

Phenylketonuria. PKU arises from a recessive gene coming from both parents. A deficiency exists that results in the child's inability to metabolize the protein phenylalanine. If undetected and untreated, phenylalanine accumulates in the child's brain. It may not be suspected until the child nears 6 months of age. Untreated PKU results in severe mental retardation. PKU occurs in approximately one in 14,000 live births. It can be detected within the first few days after birth through a simple blood test, and the child can be treated through diet control. The diet must be continued for several years. The prognosis for intellectual functioning in children who are detected and treated early is good. The prognosis worsens as the age of detection increases.

Hypothyroidism. Hypothyroidism is characterized by the inability to produce sufficient levels of thyroid hormone. It may be caused by an inherited metabolic disorder, although most cases are not inherited. Since this hormone is necessary for growth, brain development may be retarded. In most instances screening takes place for all infants in the early days of life. Oral medication can prevent the damage to brain growth caused by this condition. Hypothyroidism occurs in approximately one in 5,000 live births.

Other Metabolic Disorders

A variety of other metabolic disorders may lead to mental retardation. Galactosemia, a condition that may lead to mental retardation, is readily detected and treated through avoidance of food and drink containing galactose (milk). Maple syrup urine disease leads to death in infancy if left untreated. It may be accompanied by severe developmental delay and occurs in one in 200,000 live births. Tay-Sachs disease is characterized by degeneration of nervous tissue, blindness, deafness, severe mental retardation, and death by 5 years of age. This condition can be diagnosed prenatally, but there is no known treatment.

Other Genetic Disorders

A variety of other disorders result from genetic defects. In combination with environmental factors, the results may be moderate to severe developmental delay. One of these disorders is neurofibromatosis, a disorder characterized by skin and neural tumors. Mild impairment of intellectual function is common, with severe mental retardation rare. The incidence is approximately one in 3,300 live births. There is no treatment for this disorder other than cosmetic surgery for the tumors. The offspring of individuals with neurofibromatosis have a 50 percent chance of inheriting the disorder.

Neural tube defects are multifactorial conditions that occur in one or two per 1,000 live births. The most common form of neural tube defect is spina bifida, which results when there is incomplete fusion of the vertebral tissue. The enclosed tissue may herniate through the defect, resulting in meningocele (meninges alone) or meningomyelocele (meninges, spinal cord, and spinal roots). Spina bifida results in major physical difficulties in 80 percent of the cases. In addition, approximately 25 percent of children with spina bifida are mildly to severely retarded (Holzman, 1983). In recent years, great strides have been made in the surgical management of spina bifida.

PRENATAL AND PERINATAL FACTORS

Low Birth Weight

One of the major categories of children who are at risk of displaying developmental delay are those children with a history of neonatal medical complications. The most frequently occurring neonatal medical complication, and one that is multifactored, is low birth weight. Low birth weight is a major determinant of infant mortality as well as of developmental delay in surviving infants.

A low-birth-weight infant has been defined as any infant born weighing less than 2,500 gm (approximately 5.5 lbs). However, viewing birth weight alone as a determinant for developmental risk is insufficient. In addition to birth weight, gestational age must also be considered. Thus a particular infant may be appropriate for gestational age from a birth-weight standpoint (AGA) or may be inappropriate or small for gestational age (SGA). The term *high-risk infant* has been used to describe children who are at greater risk for neurodevelopmental delay as a result of prematurity and low birth weight.

There has been increased interest in the high-risk infant population due in large measure to the increasing survival rates as a result of intensive care nursery facilities and procedures nationwide. Table 2-1 presents survival by birth-weight categories for three time periods. Table 2-2 demonstrates the impact of neonatal intensive care on survival rates. It is obvious that survival rates for infants in the low birth-weight categories have been steadily increasing.

Increased survival rates lead directly to increased numbers of children who are subsequently at risk for displaying developmental delay. Hence, a new population of children — those who have survived a difficult neonatal period — are attracting interest from a wide variety of professionals. A look

TABLE 2-1. Survival by birth weight categories for three time periods

Birth weight (gm)/years	Number born	Number survived	Percentage survived
< 750			
1965–1969	8	0	0
1970–1975	12	1	8.3
1976–1981	27	6	22.2
750–1000			
1965–1969	26	7	26.9
1970–1975	24	6	25.0
1976–1981	77	46	59.7
1001–1250			
1965–1969	31	17	54.8
1970–1975	41	29	70.7
1976–1981	81	70	86.4
1251–1500			
1965–1969	35	21	60.0
1970–1975	51	41	80.4
1976–1981	104	97	93.3

Source: Adapted from J. Hunt, W. Tooley, and D. Harvin (1982). Learning disabilities in children with birthweights less than 1500 grams. *Seminars in Perinatology, 6,* 20. Data was collected in the San Francisco metropolitan area.

TABLE 2-2. Impact of neonatal intensive care (IC) on survival rates

	Hospital	*Before IC*	*After IC*
Neonatal mortality	St. Boniface	5.0	3.5
(0–6 days [a])	Women's College	10.6	6.2
	Jewish General	7.6	6.4
	Queens	17.0	9.9
Perinatal mortality [b]	St. Boniface	13.9	7.0
	St. Joseph's	21.6	19.0
	Women's College	20.5	14.8
	Royal Victoria	19.1	15.2
	Jewish General	20.9	14.9
	Grace	12.5	7.7

[a] Per 1,000 births.
[b] Per 1,000 births.
Source: Adapted from P. Sawyer (1981). The organization of perinatal care with particular reference to the newborn. In G. Avery (Ed.), *Neonatology, Pathophysiology and Management of the Newborn.* Philadelphia: J. B. Lippincott Co.

at the numbers of children who are at risk of developmental delay due to low birth weight and prematurity should serve to alert the practitioner to the scope of assessment activity that will ultimately be directed toward this population of children. By age 5, overall estimates of children with disabling conditions range from 8.5 to 12 percent (Healey, 1983). Many of these children will have a history of neonatal medical complications associated with low birth weight and prematurity. Tables 2-3 and 2-4 present data on the proportion of low birth-weight and very low birth-weight infants (birth weight below 1,500 gm).

A state-by-state ranking of the incidence of low birth weight is presented in Table 2-5. These data amplify the national scope of high-risk infants and their subsequent need of careful developmental monitoring. Further analysis reveals that the United States does not compare favorably with other industrialized countries in the overall percentage of low birth-weight infants born yearly (Table 2-6).

Low birth weight is associated with a variety of factors that directly bear on the developmental expectations of school-age children. A careful review of the literature associated with the developmental performance of low birth-weight infants reveals that as birth weight decreases, the amount of time that surviving infants spend in the intensive care nursery increases (Table 2-7). In addition, low birth-weight babies are more likely to require rehospitalization when compared with normal birth-weight babies (Table 2-8). Various additional statements about the increased risk seen in low birth-weight infants include the following:

**TABLE 2-3. Percentage of
low-birth-weight infants**

	1970	1980	1982	1983
All	7.9	6.8	6.8	6.8
Black	13.9	12.5	12.4	12.6
White	6.8	5.7	5.6	5.7

Source: Adapted from the National Center for Health
Statistics (1985). Monthly vital statistics report, 34, 6,
Supplement, Sept. 20, 1985.

**TABLE 2-4. Incidence of very-low-
birth-weight infants (< 1,500 gm)**

	1982		1983	
	Number	Percentage	Number	Percentage
All	43,212	1.17	43,161	1.17
White	27,007	0.9	26,872	0.9
Nonwhite	16,205	2.19	16,289	2.54

Source: Adapted from the National Center for Health Statistics (1985).
Monthly vital statistics report, 34, 6, Supplement, Sept. 20, 1985.

1. Low birth weight is strongly associated with infant morbidity, including congenital malformation and retardation (Hutchins, Kessel, and Placek, 1984).
2. For infants who do not die in the first year of life, low birth weight
   is associated with developmental disabilities, cerebral palsy, and
   other handicaps (President's Committee on Mental Retardation,
   1980).
3. More than 60 percent of all deaths in the neonatal period (first 28
   days of life), and 20 percent of deaths between 28 days and 1 year,
   are of low birth-weight babies (Committee to Study the Prevention
   of Low Birthweight, 1985).
4. Low birth-weight babies have a 40 times greater risk of death in
   the neonatal period; very low birth-weight babies have a risk of
   death 200 times greater than babies born weighing more than
   2,500 gm (Committee to Study the Prevention of Low Birthweight,
   1985).

TABLE 2-5. Babies born under 2,500 gm ranked by state

Rank	State	Total percentage	Rank	State	Total percentage
1	Alaska	4.7	26	Kentucky	6.9
1	Arizona	4.7	26	Texas	6.9
1	North Dakota	4.7	29	Hawaii	7.0
4	Iowa	5.0	29	Michigan	7.0
4	Oregon	5.0	29	Nevada	7.0
6	Minnesota	5.1	32	Wyoming	7.1
6	New Hampshire	5.1	33	Delaware	7.2
6	South Dakota	5.1	33	Illinois	7.2
9	Washington	5.2	33	New York	7.2
10	Nebraska	5.4	33	New Jersey	7.2
10	Wisconsin	5.4	33	Virginia	7.2
11	Idaho	5.6	33	Washington, DC	7.2
11	Maine	5.6	39	Florida	7.4
11	Montana	5.6	40	New Mexico	7.6
11	Utah	5.6	41	Maryland	7.7
16	Massachusetts	5.9	42	Arkansas	7.8
16	Vermont	5.9	42	California	7.8
18	Kansas	6.1	42	North Carolina	7.8
19	Indiana	6.3	45	Alabama	7.9
20	Connecticut	6.4	45	Colorado	7.9
20	Rhode Island	6.4	47	Tennessee	8.0
22	Missouri	6.7	48	Georgia	8.4
22	Ohio	6.7	49	Louisiana	8.6
22	Oklahoma	6.7	49	South Carolina	8.6
22	Pennsylvania	6.7	51	Mississippi	8.8
22	West Virginia	6.7			

Source: Adapted from the National Center for Health Statistics (1985). Monthly vital statistics report, 34, 6, Supplement, Sept. 20, 1985.

5. Very low birth-weight babies (< 1,500 gm) account for 25 to 30 percent of deaths between 28 days and 1 year (McCormack, 1985).
6. Low birth weight is the major determinant of neonatal mortality, even after controlling for other risk factors (McCormack, 1985).

TABLE 2-6. Low birth-weight ranking of the United States compared with other countries with low infant mortality*

Rank	Country	Low birth weight (%)
1	Sweden	3.6
2	Finland	3.9
3	The Netherlands	4.0
4	Norway	4.2
5	New Zealand	4.9
6	Austria	5.0
7	Japan	5.1
8	Australia	5.8
9	Czechoslovakia	6.1
10	Israel	6.3
11	German Democratic Republic	6.3
12	Canada	6.4
13	Denmark	6.4
14	France	6.5
15	Federal Republic of Germany	6.7
16	United Kingdom	7.0
17	United States	7.4

* Low infant mortality is defined as 25 per 1,000 live births or less.
Source: Adapted from The State of the World's Children (1985).
United Nations Children's Fund, p. 115.

TABLE 2-7. Mean days in neonatal intensive care for surviving infants

Birth weight status (gm)	Days in nursery
Above 2,500	3.5
2,001–2,500	7.0
1,501–2000	24.0
Below 1,500	57.0
Below 1,000	89.0

Source: Adapted from the Committee to Study the Prevention of Low Birthweight (1985). *Preventing low birth weight.* Washington, DC: Institute of Medicine.

**TABLE 2-8. Rehospitalization of babies
in their first year by weight (1980)**

Birth weight status (gm)	Percentage hospitalized	Length of stay (days)
Very low birth weight (< 1,500)	40.0	16.0
Low birth weight (< 2,500)	19.0	12.5
Normal (> 2,500)	8.7	8.9

Source: Adapted from the Committee to Study the Prevention of Low Birthweight (1985). *Preventing low birth weight.* Washington, DC: Institute of Medicine.

7. Very low birth-weight infants are at serious risk of disabilities. Forty-two percent will have some neurologic handicap or congenital anomaly, with 14 percent severely affected, compared with 19 percent and 2 percent, respectively, of normal birth-weight infants (McCormack, 1985).
8. Premature low birth-weight infants are 10 times more likely to be mentally retarded than normal infants (President's Committee on Mental Retardation, 1980).

For a more complete discussion of the increased developmental risk observed in low-birth-weight infants, see Rossetti, 1986; Davies and Tizard, 1975; Ellison, 1984; Manser, 1984; and Noble–Jamieson, Lukeman, Silverman, and Davies, 1982.

Inadequate Prenatal Care

Prenatal care is usually defined in numeric terms. That is, inadequate prenatal care means no medical care before delivery, medical care starting after the first or second trimester of pregnancy, or not enough prenatal visits (usually eight or nine visits depending on the length of the pregnancy). A variety of investigators have reported that inadequate prenatal care increases the risk of neonatal and perinatal death and low birth weight (Lewit, 1983; Gortmaker, 1979; Showstack, Budetti, and Minkler, 1984; Eisner, 1979). The relationship of low birth weight and prematurity to mental retardation is obvious; hence, the issue of inadequate prenatal care should be of concern to the practitioner when deciding which children might require early childhood assessment activity. Various programs to increase the amount of prenatal care to those women who are at increased risk of receiving inadequate prenatal care have shown promising results. The result is that improving the quantity and quality of prenatal care does lead to reductions in preterm births, in low birth-weight infants, and, by inference, in developmental disabilities. This has been incorporated into national goals set by the U.S. Surgeon General. The Surgeon General has set 1990 as a target date by which the proportion of women in any county or racial or ethnic group who obtain no prenatal care during the first trimester of pregnancy be no larger than 10 percent (National Center for Health Statistics, 1983).

Strobino (1986) studied national and state trends regarding the adequacy of prenatal care. Strobino's results indicate that although the percentage of women taking advantage of early prenatal care increased sharply between 1970 and 1980, the percentage leveled off between 1981 and 1983. In fact, for some segments of the population (e.g., minority women) the 1981 to 1983 period showed a reversal. Because sufficient prenatal care is related to prevention of factors that might contribute to developmental disability, this issue should be of concern to the infant-toddler assessor.

Maternal Nutrition

Lack of adequate maternal nutrition has been known for a long time to contribute adversely to fetal health and development. Both maternal malnutrition and malnutrition in early life are related to various aspects of developmental pathology. Maternal malnutrition is related to low birth weight, prematurity, stunted growth patterns, retardation of brain development, cognitive deficiencies, and behavioral problems. Many studies have described in great detail the connection between malnutrition and mental development as well as between learning and behavioral problems (Rush, 1984). Huber (1983) notes positive correlations between malnutrition and reduced IQ scores, motor behavior deficits, behavior development, and school performance. Evidence indicates that children who were nutritionally deprived and who have been given nutritional supplementation show increased attention and alertness. One interesting finding of such studies has been that minimal recovery of malnourished children is noted following nutritional supplementation in children who did not receive increased cognitive stimulation, with near-normal performance being present in malnourished children who received both increased cognitive stimulation and nutritional rehabilitation (Rush, 1984).

In investigations concerned with nutrition, it is quite difficult to determine to what extent lower developmental performance and other developmental problems in later life were due to prenatal or neonatal nutritional deprivation or to a combination of other social and cultural variables. The social context in which a lack of sufficient nutritional support is likely to be noted also contributes to the areas of deficit previously noted.

Adolescent Pregnancy

As a group, adolescent women are at greater risk for infant mortality, premature births, low birth-weight infants, and complications of labor and delivery that frequently accompany neurologic defects in their infants. Age alone is not the single most important factor when considering adolescent pregnancy (except for those women under 16 years). It appears that other attributes of teenage women who have babies (e.g., poor nutrition, low income, lack of education, inadequate prenatal care) explain the increased risk associated with adolescent pregnancy.

Infants born to adolescent women are at far greater risk of low birth weight. For example, in 1978, 17 percent of all births were to teenagers, yet 24 percent of all low birth-weight infants had a teenage mother (Loman, 1986). In 1983 alone, 47,500 low birth-weight infants were born to women under 20 years of age. There has been little or no reduction in low birth weight among teenage mothers since 1978. Table 2-9 presents data on the percentage of low birth weight by age of mother. Adolescent mothers also tend to suffer more from anemia during pregnancy than do mothers over 20 years of age. Teenage mothers have a higher rate of toxemia as well (Makinson, 1985).

In addition to the medical correlates of teenage pregnancy, various other factors must be considered when viewing the potential for developmental pathology. The child-rearing context for children of teenage mothers is likely to be a source of problems as well. Teenage mothers finish high school less often. They have higher unemployment rates, and a significant percentage of teenage mothers are unmarried. Those who are married show a higher percentage of divorce (Select Committee on Children, Youth, and Families, 1986). Baldwin and Cain (1980) have shown that

TABLE 2-9. Percentage of low birth-weight infants (less than 2,500 gm) based on maternal age

Maternal age (yr)	Percentage		
	1978	1980	1983
Under 15	14.3	14.6	14.5
15–19	9.9	9.9	9.4
20–24	7.1	6.9	7.0
25–29	6.0	5.8	5.9

Source: Adapted from the Children's Defense Fund (1986). *Maternal-child health data book.* Washington, DC: Department of Health and Human Services.

children who live alone with their teenage mothers are generally in poorer
physical health than comparable children who live in a more stable environment. They are more likely to show cognitive deficits. There is also a
greater likelihood that children born to adolescent mothers will be abused
or neglected (Makinson, 1985). Children born to teenagers are more likely
to be injured or hospitalized by the age of 5 (Digest, 1984). This may not be
due directly to the youth of the mother when the child was born but to her
associated deficits in education and income and to the greater likelihood of
marital breakup (Loman, 1986, p. 24).

Maternal Substance Abuse

Alcohol Abuse. Alcohol and a number of other chemicals that the mother
may ingest during pregnancy are known teratogens. These can damage the
fetus's physical growth and, later in life, the child's psychological growth.
These teratogens can not only cause congenital defects but may be responsible for functional deficiencies later in life.

Numerous studies link alcohol consumption during pregnancy with birth
defects. Alcohol interferes with the fetus's ability to receive sufficient oxy-
gen and nourishment for normal cell development in the brain and in other
developing body organs.

Mills (1984) collected data on over 31,000 pregnancies. Results indicated that the consumption of two drinks daily was associated with a substantially increased risk of producing a growth-retarded infant. The results
of alcohol consumption during pregnancy run on a continuum. At the mild
end, the child may be born with a slight reduction in birth weight. At the
extreme end, the result may be severe deformity or fetal death. *Fetal alcohol syndrome* (FAS) is the diagnostic term used to describe those children
born to mothers who ingested dangerous amounts of alcohol during pregnancy. FAS has been described as a combination of growth retardation,
mental retardation, and unusual physical development, including malformation of the face and various organs (Loman, 1986). Streissguth and La Due
(1985) describe a trilogy of symptoms in the FAS child: growth deficiencies, dysmorphic characteristics (minor physical anomalies), and CNS dysfunction. Heart defects occur in 30 to 40 percent of children with FAS.

Although not all FAS children are mentally retarded, the upper range of
IQs of FAS children studied has usually been close to 100. The average
range of IQ for FAS children has been 50 to 60. It is estimated that approximately 2.5 percent of FAS children are so severely retarded that they require continuous institutionalization (Harwood and Napolitano, 1985). The
full impact of alcohol on the developing fetus was expressed in 1981 when
the U.S. Surgeon General advised pregnant women not to consume any alcoholic beverages.

Smoking and Pregnancy. The adverse effects of maternal cigarette smoking are well documented and show a dose-response relationship. Growth retardation and subsequent developmental delay have been found in excess in infants of cigarette-smoking mothers. Stein and Kline (1983) reviewed a large number of studies concerning smoking and pregnancy. Their overall conclusion was that smoking during pregnancy is associated with reduction in birth weight. They concluded that reductions were in the range of 150 to 250 gm, although they were not able to specify exactly what quantity of smoking produced the effects.

Research over the past 30 years has consistently demonstrated the relationship between smoking and poor perinatal outcome. It is estimated that smoking is a significant contributing factor in 20 to 40 percent of the cases of low birth-weight infants born in the United States (Public Health Service, 1979). Furthermore, it has been demonstrated that people who breathe the smoke produced by others in the home and workplace are at increased overall health risk. The U.S. Surgeon General has estimated a smoking prevalence rate of 20 to 30 percent among pregnant women in the United States (Public Health Service, 1980).

Prescription Drugs. Surprisingly few prescription drugs are known teratogens, and those that are depend on dose, route, and timing of administration and, presumably, on the genotype of the mother and infant for their teratogenicity. Several of the prescription drugs that are known teratogens bear discussion.

Thalidomide has a known adverse effect on the fetus at critical periods during fetal development. More than 90 percent of infants whose mothers received the drug between 34 and 50 days' gestation had major malformations, the most striking of which was profound disruption of limb development. Anomalies of eyes, ears, teeth, and intestine were also present in some infants.

Folic acid antagonists, warfarin, and some *anticonvulsants* are known teratogens. If a pregnant woman ingests these drugs during crucial stages of fetal development, the infant may be born with hydrocephalus, craniosynostosis, limb abnormalities, mental deficiency, hypothyroidism, hypoplasia of the nose, shortened digits, neural tube defects, skeletal abnormalities, cleft lip, and cardiac defects (Meadow, 1968). Organic mercury, tetracycline, large doses of vitamin A, and androgenic hormones have also been linked with a variety of adverse effects on the fetus.

Illegal Drugs. In many instances users of illegal drugs are using multiple drugs; hence, the evaluation of the effect of a given drug becomes complex. Prematurity, low birth weight for gestational age, and perinatal asphyxia are more common among abusers of drugs (Avery and First, 1989). In addition, adverse effects during pregnancy include spontaneous abortion, abruptio placentae, and stillbirth. Two street drugs that are known to have adverse effects on the developing fetus are cocaine and heroin.

Use of cocaine by women in the child-bearing years has increased dramatically in the 1980s (Avery and First, 1989). Infants whose mothers used cocaine during pregnancy are reported to be hypertonic and irritable and have depressed interactive behaviors. Complications of pregnancy including abruptio placentae occur at a higher rate in cocaine abusers than in the general pouplation. The rate of congenital malformations is higher in cocaine abusers (Bingol, Fuchs, and Diaz, 1987).

Maternal heroin injection is associated with evidence of fetal distress, including low birth weight. Infants may display severe withdrawal symptoms 24 to 72 hours after birth. These infants are hyperactive and, if severely affected, may have seizures. Tachycardia, vomiting, diarrhea, and fever may appear during the withdrawal period. Irritability and jitteriness may persist for a month or longer.

Maternal Infection and Diseases

A variety of maternal diseases can affect fetal well-being. One such disease is diabetes mellitus, a chronic disease. It cannot always be detected before pregnancy. However, if previously present, diabetes is exacerbated by the pregnancy. Infants born to diabetic mothers may display heart defects, skeletal deformities, respiratory distress, neurologic problems, and potential convulsions (Oliphant, Geiger–Parker, and Gundell, 1985).

Several types of maternal infections can also be quite damaging to fetal development. These include rubella, toxoplasmosis, and cytomegalovirus (CMV). Rubella is a viral infection that can result in heart anomalies, cataracts, glaucoma, bone lesions, mental retardation, and deafness. Toxoplasmosis is a maternal infection that can be transmitted to the developing fetus. In approximately one in 1,000 live births the infant is born with congenital infections. Great variability exists regarding the symptoms associated with this infection. Blindness, CNS damage, jaundice, hydrocephalus, and intercranial calcifications may result. Mental retardation may also result. CMV is also an intrauterine and early postnatal infection that can damage the CNS and result in mental retardation.

POSTNATAL ENVIRONMENTAL FACTORS

The final category of factors that are significant in developmental delay are those in the child's postnatal environment. The relationship between these factors and those mentioned in previous sections is strong. It is imperative that the practitioner keep a transactional view of causation in mind when considering postnatal environmental factors. Those children who are most likely to display problems outlined in the previous sections may also display one or more of the factors specified in the following section. The practitioner must be aware of all factors that may contribute to developmental pathology and of how they interact with one another.

Environmental Poisons

There has been increasing concern in recent years regarding sources of environmental poisons that result in health hazards for children and adults alike. Environmental toxins have been implicated in increasing cancer rates as well as in less catastrophic health hazards. One source of danger for children emanates from high doses of lead in the environment. High lead levels result in serious health problems, including convulsions, coma, and even death. Chronic low-level exposure to lead is a known source of illness in children. Research has shown that younger children absorb and retain a higher percentage of lead than do adults (Zeigler, Edwards, and Jensen, 1978). Children who suffer chronic exposure to lead show impairment in general developmental performance across all developmental domains (Needleman, 1979). Prenatal exposure to elevated lead levels may also result in congenital anomalies (Needleman, 1984). Lead is known to cause neurologic damage and may result in mental retardation or at least developmental delay. Since lead is so pervasive in the human environment, it is one of the most prevalent causes of childhood health problems.

Childhood poisonings continue to be an important public health problem. Poison control centers in the United States handle over 1,500,000 poison-related calls annually, many of them concerning childhood poisoning incidents. Despite a dramatic fall in the number of childhood poisonings resulting from childproof containers, over 110,000 children under 5 years of age were treated for toxic exposures in 1983, and 14 percent of them required hospitalization. If medical help is not available, or if enough of the toxic agent is ingested, permanent damage may result. This damage may manifest itself in various degrees of developmental pathology.

Childhood Diseases

A variety of diseases are known to contribute to developmental pathology. Certainly any child who is medically fragile during the first 2 years of life is at risk for displaying patterns of delayed development. If a child is not afforded sufficient levels of environmental interaction due to repeated illness, regardless of whether the illness is serious or minor but repeated, a higher risk of developmental delay is present. Medical conditions implicated as contributing to developmental delay can be catastrophic, such as meningitis, or a series of less serious illnesses that plague the child. Meningitis is a particularly troublesome causative agent of developmental pathology. An infection of the brain lining typically occurring in infancy or early childhood, it may result in mental retardation, hearing loss, or speech and motor deficits.

Accidents and Trauma

Accidents and trauma are serious causes of disabilities in children. Trunkey (1983) indicates that physical trauma is the principal cause of death in the United States among persons 1 to 38 years of age. In 1982 there were over 300,000 cases of permanent disability resulting from trauma. Some children are seen as injury prone or injury repeaters. No single definition of an injury-repeating or accident-prone child has been fully accepted by the medical community. Some physicians consider a child with two or more injuries requiring medical attention within a 12-month period to be an injury repeater. For most types of childhood injuries, boys outnumber girls across all age ranges and socioeconomic groups. Injuries may also be sorted by age and developmental considerations. For example, the peak age range for childhood poisoning occurs at 18 to 36 months, whereas for bicycle injuries it is 5 to 8 years.

According to Avery and First (1989), families of injury repeaters may be more disorganized and socially isolated than are others. They are often under considerable daily stress, and the injuries often occur around peak times of distraction when supervision of the children may be minimal. In many instances the physical environment of the injured child may be unsafe. For children, various types of trauma may result in cerebral palsy, mental retardation, or a variety of other developmental pathologies.

Early Experience and Education

It is widely accepted that environmental factors can be as detrimental to developmental progress as biologic factors. Thus, children who are receiving inadequate early experience are certainly at risk for displaying later patterns of developmental deviancy. If the practitioner keeps in mind the transactional manner of viewing the interaction between the environment and the child's constitution, a more complete understanding of the manner in which these factors affect one another is possible.

The general quality of experiences afforded the infant or toddler directly affects developmental progress. Inadequate early experience and impoverished parent-child interaction are certainly implicated as contributing to developmental delay. Bijou (1983) has noted that the mother's involvement with her infant is the most consistent predictor of scores on developmental scales. He goes on to note that infants who have received less verbal and social attention from their mothers tend to score lower on IQ tests. On the other hand, children who display increased levels of verbal fluency tend to be the products of families that demonstrate high verbal interaction between infants and mothers (Jones, 1972).

There is a wide range of quality regarding the early experiences afforded infants and toddlers. On one end of the continuum are caregiver-child relationships that are nurturing and purposefully geared to enhance infant development. On the other end are homes in which nurturing is not a priority and in which neglect and abuse may be the norm. Factors previously mentioned in this chapter are known to contribute to the increased possibility of abuse and neglect (e.g., prematurity, extended periods of mother-child separation, extended periods of child illness in infancy, mental retardation, and physical handicaps) and are overrepresented in the populations of children who are receiving less than optimal nurturing in the home setting.

Sociocultural and Economic Factors

One significant supposition that has been consistently pointed out in the information discussed thus far is that developmental disabilities do not depend on independent causes but rather on interacting biologic, social, and cultural factors. Even when biologic etiologies appear to be of central importance, these physical causes are set in a social and cultural context and are subject to the many determinants present there.

Bijou (1983) has estimated that 80 to 85 percent of the cases of developmental disability may be termed sociocultural. What is clear is that sociocultural factors contribute significantly to developmental delay. It is imperative that the practitioner keep this in mind as assessment and intervention services are provided to infants and toddlers and their families. Many of the topics discussed thus far appear in greater frequency in settings in which economic conditions and sociocultural status are not optimal. Several of these are amplified below.

Low Birth Weight. Low birth weight is associated with low socioeconomic status as measured by social class, income, and education. The single most important predictor of infant survival continues to be birth weight (Hogue, Buehler, Strauss, and Smith, 1987). Two-thirds of infant deaths in 1980 occurred during the neonatal period. Of those, more than half occurred to infants weighing less than 1,500 gm. Those infants, who comprise less than 1 percent of all live births, account for almost 40 percent of all infant deaths (Hogue, Buehler, Strauss, and Smith, 1987). Infants who are the products of very low socioeconomic environments are certainly at increased risk for low birth weight and the resultant complications associated with it.

Maternal Education. Infant mortality declines with increasing maternal education across racial groups. The decline, however, is steeper for infants born to white women. The relationship between socioeconomic status and educational level is a strong one and certainly must be considered a contributing factor to developmental disability. Table 2-10 presents data regarding infant mortality by race and level of maternal education.

Prenatal Care. The link between socioeconomic status and securing adequate prenatal care is obvious. Infants born to mothers who obtained prenatal care beginning in the first trimester experienced substantially fewer complications in the neonatal period. Women of lower socioeconomic status seek less medical attention in general and seek prenatal care at a lower rate and at less optimal times. More than 5 percent of all pregnant women receive prenatal care only in the third trimester of pregnancy or not at all, and this percentage has been increasing, rather than diminishing, since 1981. The percentage of nonwhite women is more than double that for white women (National Center for Health Statistics, 1983).

Adolescent Pregnancy. In 1980, there were 562,330 babies born in the United States to teenage mothers (19 years of age or under). The offspring of teenage mother have long been known to be at increased risk of infant mortality and developmental pathology largely because many weigh less than 2,500 gm. Disadvantaged socioeconomic groups and racial minorities are overrepresented in the population of teenage mothers (Friede et al., 1987). Table 2-11 presents information on infant mortality risk per 1,000 live births by race and age. Note that the factors contributing greatly to infant mortality are the identical factors the practitioner is concerned with for the presence of developmental pathology for surviving infants.

TABLE 2-10. Infant mortality risk per 1,000 live births based on maternal race and level of education

Maternal education (yr)	Race (%)		
	Black	White	Total
0–8	25.6	15.1	17.2
9–11	22.5	13.7	16.3
12	18.1	8.9	10.6
13–15	16.2	7.4	7.3
Above 16	13.6	6.7	7.3

Source: Adapted from C. Hogue, J. Buehler, L. Strauss, & J. Smith (1987). Overview of the national infant mortality survey (NIMS) project: Design, methods, and results. *Public Health Reports, 102,* 126.

TABLE 2-11. Infant mortality per 1,000
live births by maternal age and race

Maternal age (yr)	Race (%)		
	Black	White	Total
10–14	36.0	25.0	31.5
15–19	21.2	13.6	15.8
20–24	18.5	9.4	11.1

Source: Adapted from C. Hogue, J. Buehler, L. Strauss, and J. Smith
(1987). Overview of the national infant mortality survey (NIMS)
project: Design, methods, and results. *Public Health Reports,
102,* 126.

Overall, children of teenage mothers are more likely to be abused or neglected, to suffer injuries and hospitalization, and to be in poorer physical
health. These problems are due less to the mother's biologic youth than to
the economic adversity that is a correlate of teenage pregnancy (Loman,
1986). Burden and Klerman (1984) and Sidel (1986) conclude that most
teenage mothers are single and poor, with 60 percent receiving welfare at
some time. Education is interrupted by the pregnancy and birth, and day
care is unavailable. Thus, the teenage mother remains uneducated, un-
skilled, unemployed, and often unemployable. The outcome is continuing
poverty. The fundamental problem of teenage mothers, therefore, is that
adolescent mothers as a group remain poor and powerless.

Miscellaneous Factors. Several additional factors must be considered
when viewing socioeconomic correlates of developmental disability.

Maternal infections are more prevalent in the underprivileged population. CMV infection in pregnant women can cause malformations in the
fetal brain. The virus is associated with younger females, low socioeconomic status, and crowded living conditions (Taft, 1980).

Children who are poorer and who live in urban areas are more likely to
be exposed to lead poisoning. As Loman (1986) has stated, "black children
from families earning less than $6,000 per year have dangerous blood lead
levels with a prevalence of 18.6 percent as compared with 3.9 percent for
the general population."

Nersesian (1985) indicated that children from low-income families are
2.6 times as likely to die of accidental injury than are other children. The relationship between low-income families and serious accidents of children is
easy to understand. Substandard and unsafe housing, unsafe appliances,
homes with increased susceptibility to fire, poorer fire protection, lack of
funds to purchase car safety seats, and increased numbers of children of

poor families who are left alone in the home also contribute to increased mortality and morbidity due to accident.

Serious illnesses in children are also more prevalent in lower-income families. Zill (1980) has indicated that low-income children are more likely to suffer from chronic conditions that interfere with schoolwork. Starfield and Egbuonu (1982) indicate that hearing deficits, vision disorders, psychological problems, and iron deficiency and anemia occur in greater frequency in low-income families.

SUMMARY

An enormous array of handicapping conditions and their causes exist. Hayden and Beck (1982) estimate that there are 500 different anomalies associated with mental retardation, over 4,000 separate causes of severe handicaps, and over 200 recognizable patterns of malformations in children. This multitude of conditions is only summarized in this chapter. The onset of developmental problems may occur at any time during the three major developmental periods: prenatal, perinatal, and postnatal. Bricker lists nine separate categories for conceptualizing causes of developmental pathology in infant and toddlers (1986, p. 141). These are:

1. Infections (e.g., meningitis)
2. Intoxication (e.g., poisoning)
3. Accident or trauma (e.g., head injury)
4. Metabolic disorders (e.g., PKU)
5. CNS disorders (e.g., tumor)
6. Chromosomal disorders (e.g., Down syndrome)
7. Gestational disorders (e.g., prematurity)
8. Psychosocial disorders (e.g., environmental deprivation)
9. Unknown (e.g., no overt causal factors)

The infant-toddler assessor must be familiar with concepts surrounding causation. This information will help in determining the recipients of infant-toddler assessment, interpreting assessment results, communicating those results to other professionals, and suggesting intervention strategies. The categories of causative factors discussed in this chapter in large measure answer the question, "Who are the recipients of infant-toddler assessment?" The assessor must realize, however, that any classification system, although helpful, has some imperfections. Any categorization paradigm used by the assessor must be employed with flexibility and common sense.

STUDY QUESTIONS

1. What are the three models of causation relative to developmental disability that were discussed in the chapter? How do they differ? What are the strengths and weaknesses of each?
2. Various prenatal and perinatal factors contribute to developmental pathology. List as many as you can, and describe how these might delay normal development.
3. Developmental disabilities associated with postnatal factors are also important in developmental delay. Describe these postnatal factors, and discuss how they might delay development.

REFERENCES

Avery, M., & First, L. (1989). *Pediatric medicine*. Baltimore: Williams & Wilkins.

Baldwin, W., & Cain, V. (1980). The children of teen parents. *Family Planning Perspectives, 12*, 34.

Bingol, N., Fuchs, M., & Diaz, V. (1987). Teratogenicity of cocaine in humans. *Journal of Pediatrics, 110*, 93.

Bijou, S. (1983). The prevention of mild and moderate retarded development. In F. Menolascino (Ed.), *Curative aspects of mental retardation*. Baltimore: Brooks Publishing.

Bricker, D. (1986). *Early education of at risk and handicapped infants, toddlers, and preschool children*. Glenview, IL: Scott Foresman.

Bronfenbrenner, U. (1975). Nature with nurture: A reinterpretation of the evidence. In A. Montague (Ed.), *Race and IQ*. New York: Oxford University Press.

Bruner, J. (1978). From communication to language: A psychosocial perspective. In I. Markoiva (Ed.), *The social context of language*. London: Wiley.

Burden, D., & Klerman, L. (1984). Teenage parenthood: Factors that lessen economic dependence. *Social Work, 11*, 16.

Children's Defense Fund. (1986). *Maternal-child health data book*. Washington, DC: Department of Health and Human Services.

Committee to Study the Prevention of Low Birthweight. (1985). *Preventing low birth weight*. Washington, DC: Institute of Medicine.

Davies, P., & Tizard, J. (1975). Very low birth weight and subsequent neurological defect. *Developmental Medicine and Child Neurology, 17*, 3.

Digest. (1984). Children born to teens are more likely to be injured or hospitalized by age 5. *Family Planning Perspectives, 16*, 238.

Eisner, V. (1979). The risk of low birthweight. *American Journal of Public Health, 69*, 887.

Ellison, P. (1984). Neurological development of the high-risk infant. *Clinics in Perinatology, 11*, 1.

Escalona, S. (1982). Babies at double hazard: Early development of infants at biologic and social risk. *Pediatrics, 70*, 5.

Friede, A., Baldwin, W., Rhodes, P., Buehler, J., Strauss, L., Smith, J., & Houge, C.

(1987). Young maternal age and infant mortality: The role of low birthweight. *Public Health Reports, 102,* 192.

Greenfield, P., & Smith, P. (1976). *The structure of communication in early language development.* New York: Academic Press.

Gortmaker, S. (1979). The effects of prenatal care upon the health of the newborn. *American Journal of Public Health, 69,* 653.

Harwood, H., & Napolitano, D. (1985). Economic implications of the fetal alcohol syndrome. *Alcohol Health and Research World, 10,* 1.

Hayden, A., & Beck, G. (1982). The epidemiology of high-risk and handicapped infants. In C. Ramey & P. Trohanis (Eds.), *Finding and educating high-risk and handicapped infants.* Baltimore: University Park Press.

Healey, A. (1983). *The needs of children with disabilities: A comprehensive view.* Iowa City: University of Iowa Press.

Heath, S. (1983). *Ways with words: Language, life and work in communities and classrooms.* Cambridge: Cambridge University Press.

Hogue, C., Buehler, J., Strauss, L., & Smith, J. (1987). Overview of the national infant mortality survey (NIMS) project: Design, methods, and results. *Public Health Reports, 102,* 126.

Holzman, N. (1983). Prenatal screening for neural tube defects. *Pediatrics, 71,* 249.

Hubbell, R. (1981). *Children's language disorders: An integrated approach.* Englewood Cliffs, NJ: Prentice-Hall.

Huber, A. (1983). Nutrition and mental retardation. In J. Matson & J. Mulick (Eds.), *Handbook of mental retardation.* New York: Pergamon Press.

Hunt, J., Tooley, W., & Harvin, D. (1982). Learning disabilities in children with birthweights less than 1500 grams. *Seminars in Perinatology, 6,* 20.

Hutchins, V., Kessel, S., & Placek, P. (1984). Trends in maternal and infant health factors associated with low birth weight, United States, 1972 and 1980. *Public Health Reports* (official journal of the US Public Health Service), *99,* 2.

Jones, P. (1982). Home environment and the development of verbal ability. *Child Development, 43,* 1081.

Lewit, E. (1983). The demand for prenatal care and the production of healthy infants. In D. Salkever (Ed.), *Research in human capital development.* Greenwich, CT: JAI Press.

Loman, T. (1986). *Prevention of developmental disabilities: The status of programs in Missouri.* Unpublished manuscript.

Manser, J. (1984). Growth in the high risk infant. *Clinics in Perinatology, 11,* 19.

Makinson, C. (1985). The health consequences of teenage pregnancy. *Family Planning Perspectives, 17,* 1985.

McCormack, M. (1985). The contribution of low birth weight to infant mortality and childhood morbidity. *New England Journal of Medicine, 2,* 312.

Meadow, S. (1968). Anticonvulsant drugs and congenital abnormalities. *Lancet, 2,* 1296.

Melcick, M. (1980). Drugs as etiologic agents in mental retardation and other developmental anomalies of the central nervous system. In M. McCormack (Ed.), *Prevention of mental retardation and other developmental disabilities.* New York: Marcel Dekker.

Menyuk, P. (1971). *The acquisition and development of language.* Englewood Cliffs, NJ: Prentice-Hall.

Mills, J. (1984). Maternal alcohol consumption and birth weight: How much drinking during pregnancy is safe? *Journal of the American Medical Association, 252,* 1875.

National Center for Health Statistics. (1985). *Monthy Vital Statistics Report, 34,* 6, Supplement, Sept. 20, 1985.

National Center for Health Statistics. (1983). *Health and prevention profile, United*

States, 1983. Hyattsville, MD: Department of Health and Human Services.

Nersesian, W. (1985). Childhood death and poverty: A study of all childhood deaths in Maine. *Pediatrics, 75,* 41.

Noble–Jamieson, C., Lukeman, D., Silverman, M., & Davies, P. (1982). Low birth weight children at school age: Neurological, psychological, and pulmonary function. *Seminars in Perinatology, 6,* 4, 266.

Needleman, H. (1979). Deficits in psychologic and classroom performance of children with elevated dentine lead levels. *New England Journal of Medicine, 300,* 689.

Needleman, H. (1984). The relationship between prenatal exposure to lead and congenital anomalies. *Journal of the American Medical Association, 251,* 22.

Oliphant, P., Geiger–Parker, B., & Gundell, G. (1985). *Programs for preventing the causes of mental retardation.* Unpublished manuscript.

Public Health Service. (1979). *Healthy people* (The Surgeon General's report on health promotion and disease prevention). Washington, DC: Department of Health and Human Services.

Public Health Service. (1980). *The health consequences of smoking for women* (a report of the Surgeon General). Washington, DC: Department of Health and Human Services.

President's Committee on Mental Retardation. (1980). *Mental retardation: Prevention strategies that work.* Washington, DC: US Department of Health and Human Services.

Pueschel, M., & Thuline, H. (1983). Chromosome disorders. In J. Matson & J. Malick (Eds.), *Handbook of mental retardation.* New York: Pergamon Press.

Ramey, C., Trohanis, P., & Hostler, S. (1982). An introduction. In C. Ramey & P. Trohanis (Eds.), *Finding and educating high risk and handicapped infants.* Baltimore, MD: University Park Press.

Rossetti, L. (1986). *High risk infants: Identification, assessment, and intervention.* Austin, TX: PRO-ED.

Rush, D. (1984). *National evaluation of the special supplemental food program for women, infants and children (WIC).* Washington, DC: Department of Agriculture.

Sameroff, A. (1975). Early influences on development: Fact or fancy? *Merrill Palmer Quarterly, 21,* 267.

Sameroff, A., & Chandler, M. (1975). Reproductive risk and the continuum of caretaking casualty. In F. Horowitz (Ed.), *Review of child development research: Vol. 4.* Chicago: University of Chicago Press.

Sawyer, P. (1981). The organization of perinatal care with particular reference to the newborn. In G. Avery (Ed.), *Neonatology, pathophysiology and management of the newborn.* Philadelphia: J.B. Lippincott Co.

Select Committee on Children, Youth, and Families. (1986). *Teen pregnancy: What is being done? A state by state look.* Washington, DC: U.S. House of Representatives, Ninety-Ninth Congress.

Showstack, J., Budetti, P., & Minkler, D. (1984). Factors associated with birthweight: An exploration of the roles of prenatal care and length of gestation. *American Journal of Public Health, 74,* 1003.

Sidel, R. (1986). *Women and children last.* New York: Viking.

Skeels, H. (1966). Adult status of children with contrasting early life experiences. *Monographs of the Society for Research in Child Development, 31,* 105.

Starfield, B., & Egbuonu, L. (1982). Child health and social status. *Pediatrics, 69,* 550.

Stein, Z., & Klein, J. (1983). Smoking, alcohol, and reproduction. *American Journal of Public Health, 73,* 1154.

Streissguth, A., & La Due, R. (1985). Psychological and behavioral effects in children prenatally exposed to alcohol. *Alcohol Health and Research World, 10,* 1.

Strobino, D. (1986). The impact of the Mississippi improved child health project on prenatal care and low birthweight. *American Journal of Public Health, 76,* 274.

Taft, L. (1980). An overview of the etiology of mental retardation and developmental disabilities. In M. McCormack (Ed.), *Prevention of mental retardation and other developmental disabilities.* New York: Marcel Dekker.

Trunkey, D. (1983). Trauma. *Scientific American, 249,* 28.

United Nation's Children's Fund. (1985). The state of the world's children. New York: Author.

Werner, E., Bierman, J., & French, F. (1971). *The children of Kauai.* Honolulu: University of Hawaii Press.

Whitehurst, G., Novak, G., & Zorn, G. (1972). Delayed speech studied in the home. *Developmental Psychology, 7,* 169.

Ziegler, E., Edwards, B., & Jensen, R. (1978). Absorption and retention of lead by infants. *Pediatric Research, 12,* 29.

Zill, N. (1980). *The state of American children according to their parents and teachers: National survey for children.* Washington, DC: Foundation for Child Development.

CHAPTER   3

Models for Infant-Toddler Assessment

Service Delivery Approach:
Team Concept
   Multidisciplinary Model
   Interdisciplinary Model
   Transdisciplinary Model

Team Management Issues

Case Management System

Settings for Infant-Toddler
Assessment
   Home Setting
   Center-Based Assessment

Professionals Involved in
Infant-Toddler Assessment
   Physician
   Physical Therapist
   Occupational Therapist
   Speech-Language Pathologist
     and Audiologist
   Nurse
   Psychologist
   Social Worker
   Early Childhood Education
     Specialist

Models for Early Casefinding

Model Systems

Summary

Study Questions

References

Once the practitioner is familiar with the populations of children at risk of displaying developmental pathology, the next course of action involves determining the most efficacious manner of delivering early intervention services. Because this text focuses on assessment and not intervention, the following discussion is directed toward the delivery of services to infants and toddlers from the assessment point of view. Although the following principles are applicable to intervention as well, this chapter is geared specifically toward describing various models of delivering infant and toddler assessment.

As increased interest is directed toward monitoring developmental progress in infants and toddlers, it is clear that many similarities exist among the several professional disciplines with expertise in child development. Because of these shared interests, which cross disciplinary lines, professionals are designing strategies to work together effectively in assessing handicapped infants and toddlers. Involvement of a wide variety of professionals is no longer just an option, since federal legislation mandates involvement of this nature.

Questions therefore arise on the most efficacious way to deliver assessment activity. Who should be involved? How should these professionals work together? How should their shared interests be coordinated? Where should their services be delivered. Chapter 3 is designed to address these issues.

SERVICE DELIVERY APPROACH: TEAM CONCEPT

The team approach to health care in general is an outgrowth of the rapid expansion of knowledge in health-related areas since World War II. As medicine became more complex, the overall number of professionals involved at some level in health-related services rapidly expanded. Thus, the number and types of health personnel grew and continues to do so today. Because of this expansion, the term *allied health professional* was coined. This term applies to a wide variety of discipines that contribute in one way or another to the array of health-related services afforded to persons in need.

The value of approaching health-related issues from a team standpoint is obvious. The specialist working alone runs the risk of developing professional "tunnel vision." A more complete discussion of the professionals involved in infant and toddler assessment, and hence members of the assessment team, will be presented later is this chapter.

As new fields of service provision developed, each discipline sought to establish its own identity and area of expertise. As a result, accreditation, certification, licensure, and registration in various fields evolved. These external regulatory mechanisms were instituted to ensure a high quality of performance by professionals in each specific discipline. One negative by-product of the carving out of specific areas of responsibility by various disciplines was a division of labor in overall service delivery. Thus, health care became highly specialized. In some instances the result was "a confusing array of technical and professional personnel working in compartmentalized tasks, often closely overlapping each other in some facet of their work and frequently out of communication with each other about the patient whom they presumably both serve" (Pellegrino, 1977, p. 27). In an effort to eliminate the "compartmentalized" delivery of services, which in effect tends to reduce overall effectiveness, the team concept was proposed.

Child development teams that were concerned with issues related to overall child health and development first appeared in the 1950s. Their number and makeup changed much over time. It was in the mid and late 1960s that refinement occurred in the delivery of intervention activity for children displaying developmental pathology. One must understand what constitutes a team to clearly understand the models of team functioning described below. Lowe and Herranen (1978) define a team as a "group of people, each of whom possess particular expertise; each of whom is responsible for making decisions; who together hold a common purpose; who meet together to communicate, collaborate, and consolidate knowledge from which plans are made, actions determined and future directions influenced" (p. 324). This definition is particularly applicable to the team concept of infant-toddler assessment regardless of the model of team functioning employed. The degree to which team members work together depends on the team's organizational model. The case manager system, which is discussed in greater detail later in this chapter, is a valuable tool to enhance communication between team members. It likewise affords greater follow-through of recommendations made by the entire team.

In addition, a rather recent concept regarding team functioning concerns the role that parents play. Current team functioning involves full participation by the parents as team members. Hence, parents are consulted, as any team member would be, regarding all decisions made for a given child, including medical management, developmental assessment issues, and long-term intervention issues.

One final comment is needed before discussing specific team organizational issues. The manner in which infant-toddler assessment is provided cannot be considered apart from an understanding of the relationship between assessment and intervention. In effect, assessment is one of the early steps taken when designing an appropriate early intervention program for a particular child. Hence, the models for assessment are quite similar to the models currently in operation to deliver early intervention services. Three general models of service delivery (team organization) will be presented: the multidisciplinary, interdisciplinary, and transdisciplinary models of infant-toddler assessment.

MULTIDISCIPLINARY MODEL

The concept of a multidisciplinary team refers to a group of individuals, from a variety of disciplines, whose efforts are discipline oriented. Although each member of the team has a common purpose and goal, an overall group effort is not required (Watkins, 1983). An example would be a situation in which a child receives separate evaluations from a number of individual professionals representing several disciplines. The results of each professional assessment are reported during a meeting of the group or through reporting on the child's records. If treatment is warranted based on the results of the evaluations, it is provided by each discipline separately with little further communication between professionals, except during regular meetings of the team to monitor the progress the child is making or to recommend further assessment. An example of an interdisciplinary team format is presented in Fig. 3-1.

On some multidisciplinary teams each team member works with a greater awareness of what other members are doing. For example, a social

FIGURE 3-1. Multidisciplinary team functioning model. Each member of the team works independently, providing services directly with little coordination or consultation. An example of this model of service delivery is a traditional hospital or clinic where children are seen consecutively by different specialists. A physician usually serves as team leader, facilitates group discussions and translates information directly to the family. (Adapted from M. Briggs [1989]. Interdisciplinary team: Goals and strategies. Paper presented at the Infants and Toddlers Communication and Intervention Workshop, Bethesda, MD.)

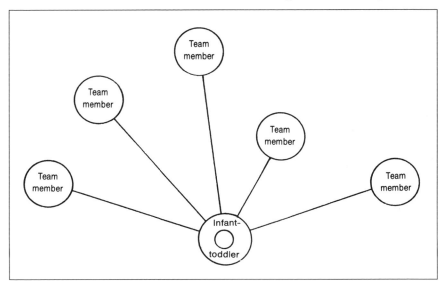

worker may take a social history. If the information suggests a problem related to feeding, then the nutritionist may be called on for a consultation.
From that point on, the speech-language pathologist or the occupational
therapist may be involved in remediating the feeding problem. As the team
continues to function, the psychologist may be involved in assessing cognitive performance. The pediatrician will likely be involved in an attempt to
confirm or rule out the presence of a medical condition contributing to the
feeding problem.

One key characteristic of the multidisciplinary team, however, is that
professional roles and responsibilities are understood and adhered to.
There is little crossing over of professional boundaries. Team functioning
such as described above can be effective. However, this mode of service
delivery does not take full advantage of the range of skills each member
brings to the problem at hand.

As Cornett and Chabon (1988) have pointed out, the multidisciplinary
team approach has received considerable support in the public sector.
Federal law mandates that a team (not necessarily the multidisciplinary
model of team functioning) approach be used in evaluating and treating
persons who participate in certain governmental programs. The Education
for All Handicapped Children Act (P.L. 94-142) as well as more recent federal legislation described in Chapter 1 mandate a team approach to assessment and intervention for infants and toddlers. The main drawback of the
multidisciplinary approach lies in the lack of full communication and
cooperative effort in assessing the child. In this model each discipline likely
sees the child, regardless of whether the child should be seen by each discipline. Each professional involved does not offer nor avail himself or herself of important observations made by other members of the assessment
team. Working together in assessing infants and toddlers can afford each
member of the team a more complete understanding of the total child
across developmental domains (Kile and Rossetti, 1989).

INTERDISCIPLINARY MODEL

In contrast to the multidisciplinary approach described above, the interdisciplinary team is characterized by a greater degree of coordination and
integration of services, which is the basic intent of early intervention activities mandated in P.L. 99-457. The law intends that disciplines work together in providing a comprehensive array of services to eligible infants and
toddlers. This is certainly more likely to occur in an interdisciplinary
model. Figure 3-2 displays an interdisciplinary team format.

Interdisciplinary teams are composed of representatives of different professions, but their activities are directed toward group-defined goals
according to individual client needs. Melvin (1980) points out that the acti-

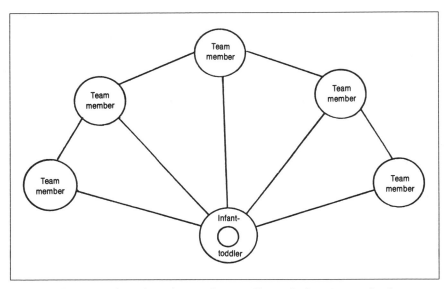

FIGURE 3-2. Interdisciplinary team format. Channels for communication among team members are clearly established. Meetings to discuss and share information are arranged. Individual team members may function independently or cooperatively in assessment and treatment planning. A case manager may be assigned to coordinate scheduling and serve as a contact person for the family. In this model, members of different disciplines commit to group decision making and development of a unified service plan. Members typically rotate responsibilities as team leader. Interactions and exchanges between disciplines are encouraged to ensure that the total needs of the child and the family are considered. (Adapted from M. Briggs. [1989]. Interdisciplinary team: Goals and strategies. Paper presented at the Infants and Toddlers Communication and Intevention Workshop, Bethesda, MD.)

vities of the interdisciplinary team involve group interaction and knowledge, which results in transferring integrated group activities into a result that is greater than the simple sum of services provided by each discipline alone. Hence, the members of the team must be aware of the need for interdependence and be willing to function in a highly integrated manner. One manner of viewing the functioning of an interdisciplinary team is presented in Table 3-1 (Cornett and Chabon, 1988).

No single model of interdisciplinary activity appears to work best. Each team that desires to work in an interdisciplinary manner must determine the method that works best given the team makeup and individual characteristics of each team member. Several guidelines should be kept in mind, however. Each member of the team must display a high level of expertise in a particular discipline. This is necessary because other team members look to one another to answer specific questions in areas of expertise outside

TABLE 3-1. Phases of interdisciplinary functioning

Data collection

Identification of roles, responsibilities, team member information needs

Data assessment

Interpretation and integration of information; diagnosis made based on contributions of each member of the team

Decision making

Options evaluated; treatment plans developed; treatment tasks assigned to team members for implementation through negotiation and consultation

Treatment

Intervention services delivered

Evaluation

Treatment process and patient outcomes evaluated; individual and collective performance of team appraised

Source: Adapted from B. Cornett & S. Chabon (1988). The clinical practice of speech-language pathology. Columbus: Merrill.

their particular domain. However, each team member must have some familiarity with other disciplines. If one views clients from the vantage point of a single discipline, the result may be tunnel vision, which undermines the purpose of the team approach. Most practitioners have been trained to perform highly specialized and independent services. As members of a team, however, professionals must be willing to relinquish a certain amount of autonomy to participate in a collaborative, interdependent effort. Without this willingness, one professional may define his or her role in a way that is incongruent with the perception of others.

Resistance to sharing information, defensiveness and "turf protection," and duplication of services result from a lack of information and poor communication among team members. Team members must make it a priority to become familiar with the skills and contributions of others, to develop interpersonal communication skills, to desire to function with high levels of collaboration and cooperation, and in many instances to compromise to guarantee effective team functioning. The bringing together of a group of child development specialists does not automatically create an effective interdisciplinary team. Attention must be given to all aspects of team functioning to ensure proper and efficacious interdisciplinary activity.

TRANSDISCIPLINARY MODEL

The distinctive characteristic of the transdisciplinary model is the crossing of traditional disciplinary boundaries by team members. This is an innovative and somewhat controversial team approach model. The term *transdisciplin-*

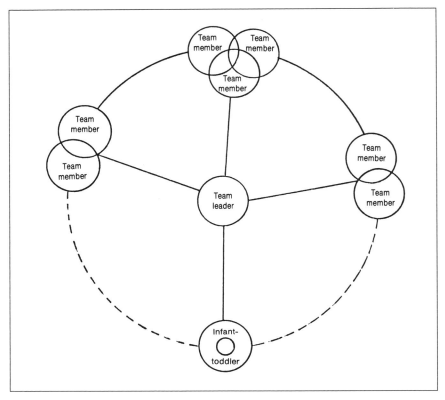

Figure 3-3. Transdisciplinary team functioning. Information, knowledge, and skills are transferred across disciplinary boundaries. The goal of this service delivery model is to seek constantly to enlarge the common core of knowledge and competencies of individual team members. Individual team members commit to teaching and learning from each other, assuming interchangeable roles and responsibilities, and allowing the needs of the child and the family to dictate the team's goals. Any member may serve as team leader. One member is typically designated as case manager and asked to translate team decisions and, in some instances, integrate the delivery of different professional services. (Adapted from M. Briggs. [1989]. Interdisciplinary team: Goals and strategies. Paper presented at the Infants and Toddlers Communication and Intervention Workshop, Bethesda, MD.)

ary was first used in 1974 to describe services provided by United Cerebral Palsy. The approach provided for a group of professionals to lend consultation and support for one professional who became the primary implementor of the services recommended by team members. Figure 3-3 outlines a transdisciplinary team functioning model.

In the transdisciplinary model each team member may be responsible for an initial assessment as well as for specific recommendations regarding treatment if indicated. Or, one team member may provide an initial assessment covering all developmental domains. Following the initial assessment, the implementation of treatment activities is assigned to a team member whose area of expertise corresponds to the individual's primary presenting area of deficit. Other team members may provide ongoing consultation to the implementor. However, the implementor is responsible for carrying out intervention recommendatons within each discipline, even though the implementor's main area of expertise is outside that of other team members. In essence the term *transdisciplinary* connotes the crossing of discipline borders and the assimilation of knowledge from other disciplines. Further, the implementor must incorporate skills and knowledge from other fields into his or her own service delivery activities. McCormick and Lee (1979) point out that the transdisciplinary approach can "broaden the sphere of influence for individual professionals because more.patients can be served that would be possible if each professional delivered separate individual treatment sessions" (p. 588).

For the transdisciplinary model to be effective, each member of the team must be committed to its implementation and value. In addition, cross-training is quite helpful. Cross-training involves specific training in transdisciplinary team functioning as well as training in areas outside one's primary area of expertise. Current financial and service delivery considerations are giving the transdisciplinary model enhanced status as a plan for delivering services that are mandated for infants and toddlers. The large team, in which each member delivers services in a multidisciplinary or interdisciplinary fashion, appears to be less practical than the transdisciplinary approach. The term *multicompetency movement* has been applied to professionals with skills in a variety of areas in addition to their primary area of expertise. The overall purpose of the multicompetency movement is to organize the task of service delivery so that more tasks can be performed without assigning a large number of specialized people (Blayney, 1986).

In an effort to expand the use of a transdisciplinary or multicompetency approach, institutions of higher learning are incorporating specific personnel preparation activities into curricula. Both the University of Alabama School of Community and Allied Health and Southern Illinois University offer skill-enhancement programs in which professionals already possessing expertise in an area can return to school to extend their knowledge and skills in related areas. In large measure, however, professionals currently operating in a transdisciplinary manner have equipped themselves through trial and error, as well as through interaction with colleagues, to function effectively in a multicompetency fashion.

The transdisciplinary approach to the delivery of infant-toddler assessment appears to be the most effective manner of providing needed assessment services to the increased numbers of children who will require such services as new federal legislation takes effect. Although cautions exist regarding its use, if implemented properly the transdisciplinary approach can be an effective and economical manner of meeting the needs of infants and toddlers who require assessment of their developmental progress.

TEAM MANAGEMENT ISSUES

Teamwork in the health care field implies that a group of people deal with an individual client. How many times have parents related that they have seen a variety of specialists regarding the needs of their child? How many times have those same parents indicated that they were frustrated because there was a lack of communication between the individual disciplines providing services to their child? What has this lack of effective communication cost the child regarding intervention effectiveness following assessment activity? Any practitioner who has gained even a moderate amount of experience providing assessment activity to infants and toddlers can relate to the sometimes common frustration of not seeing effective team functioning take place. The result is that the child suffers, and ultimately services are delivered either in a less-than-effective manner or at least at a later-than-expected date. Hence, the issue of team management is an important one for all infant-toddler assessors to understand.

Infant-toddler assessment has several components: screening and intake, the evaluation itself, the staffing, and the feedback process. To accomplish these tasks and others, there must be an effective system of team leadership in operation. A team that works well together must make a variety of decisions that relate to philosophy and the sharing of team responsibilities. The team must also make numerous day-to-day decisions that relate to the sharing of responsibilities. In large measure these practical aspects of team functioning are determined by the system of team leadership in effect. Somebody must be in charge on all teams; there is always a team leader. The leadership the team receives will in large measure determine overall team effectiveness. The team leader may be a major facilitator of teamwork, but all team members must cooperate with each other to make the assessment team function well. One noncompliant team member can cause a disruption in teamwork, thus reducing team effectiveness.

In the past it was assumed that the best leadership for infant-toddler assessment teams was provided by a physician. This style of leadership was reflected throughout the 1970s. In actual practice today, however, this is not usually the case. Many infant-toddler assessment teams today are headed by nonmedical professionals, including those functioning within a medical setting (Rossetti, 1986). At present no set format exists, nor has been postulated, for the best manner in which to select the case manager. Although the actual academic discipline of the team leader is important, other factors such as personality, the amount of time devoted to the job, and above all the degree of organizational and leadership abilities brought to the task loom large as effective team leadership is considered. These factors are in large measure independent of the person's professional identity.

CASE MANAGEMENT SYSTEM

One concept of team functioning that has gained wide acceptance is the case manager system. Holm and McCartin (1978) point out that the rationale behind the case manager system is the realization that the team approach implies that a group of people are dealing with an individual child; thus, somebody must be in charge of each case. The professional who assumes the role of being in charge for a particular child is known as the case manager. The case manager may make initial contact with the parents and, based on referral information and data gained from the parents, assign various members of the team to assess and work with the child.

In keeping with the transdisciplinary model described above, all members of the team may not need to see the child. Thus, the case manager, together with the team members who do see the child, arrive at a final disposition for each infant or toddler assessed. The decision reached by the team may involve referral for immediate early intervention, additional assessment by other team members, or simply sending the child home to be reevaluated in a specified period. If the decision involves additional assessment, the case manager arranges these appointments with the necessary team members as well as arranges staffings in which assessment results and recommendations are shared with all team members involved with the child. The case staffing gives members of the team an opportunity to discuss assessment results and to arrive at a mutual recommendation. Professional development is facilitated through a team staffing because the involvement of each team member becomes an important part of the staffing. Staffings provide an optimal setting for the exchange of observations and insights among the members of various disciplines for the benefit of the child as well as for the enlightenment and long-term education of team members.

One system that has been widely used in determining who the case manager should be is to assign manager responsibilities to the professional whose area of expertise most closely matches the primary nature of the child's problem. Thus, if the child is referred for assessment at 8 months of age, and the primary concern is a suspected delay in motor development, the physical therapist would assume case manager responsibilities. The case manager system has been shown to be an effective means of organizing service delivery when the team approach to assessment is used. If the actual number of professionals interacting with the child is low, then alternative styles of service delivery may be better suited to the model of assessment in operation.

One final comment regarding infant-toddler assessment and team involvement is needed. Cornett and Chabon (1988) ask the question, "Is there life without a team?" (p. 133). Obviously not every infant-toddler assessor has the opportunity to function in the context of a team. Many professionals do not have ready access to a comprehensive service delivery environment, while others are functioning in settings in which full access to support from other disciplines is not readily available.

An added responsibility falls on the professional who is not able to operate fully within the team context. This responsibility falls in two areas. First, the professional operating primarily alone must make every effort to become familiar with information representing a variety of disciplines to function in an interdisciplinary manner. This must be done even in the absence of regular contact with representatives of the disciplines represented on teams. If this perspective is not maintained, the professional operating alone will tend to develop a very narrow view and thus may miss important aspects of developmental delay by interpreting observed behavior from a limited professional vantage point. Second, a significant amount of initiative may be needed to devise ways to increase cooperation between professionals. This is particularly true in settings in which the basic organizational structure of service delivery is not conducive to a team approach. It is the rare professional who will not welcome initial interest by other professionals with similar interests. Initial exploratory meetings may lead to more involved discussions regarding common desires to deliver effective infant-toddler activity. Ways to facilitate regular communication can be discussed. These efforts may lead to a more open atmosphere on the part of professionals and administrators alike regarding the implementation of a team model of infant-toddler assessment. If discussions of this nature are approached from the standpoint of providing quality infant-toddler services, then a very significant common goal is shared by all. The result will more than likely be a desire to work together more effectively to provide infant-toddler assessments.

SETTINGS FOR INFANT-TODDLER ASSESSMENT

HOME SETTING

As the practitioner becomes more familiar with existing infant-toddler assessment activity, it becomes readily apparent that there are two basic environments in which services are provided: in the home setting or in a center, such as a hospital or school setting. Many models also incorporate assessment in both the home and center setting. In combination settings, the initial parent interviews may be conducted in the home, with infant-toddler assessment conducted in a center. Variations using both home and a center for infant-toddler assessment are possible depending on the unique characteristics of the agency delivering the assessment activity and the makeup of the team providing the services. Although no one setting has been deemed as "best," the practitioner must be aware of the strengths and weaknesses of each setting.

Depending on the setting in which the services are provided, various practitioners may be involved. If infant-toddler assessment is delivered in the home, the number of professionals involved will necessarily be smaller, involving as few as one or two persons. This is due to the nature of the home environment and the inability to bring a large number of team members into the home. The home assessor must be familiar with the transdisciplinary model of functioning and be trained if possible in areas outside the major area of expertise. Much present early intervention activity is delivered in the home, with very successful outcomes in many instances. Thus it is quite logical to deliver assessment services in the home setting as well. Filler (1983) lists several benefits inherent in providing infant-toddler assessment activity in the home:

1. Parents feel comfortable in their own home and therefore act more naturally.
2. Similarly, children are more likely to perform better in their own home. It affords a more naturalistic setting in which to elicit behaviors on which developmental adequacy may be judged.
3. The child's health is better protected. This may be of particular importance for those children who are medically fragile.
4. Parent and child routines are not interrupted. As a result, a more accurate sample of parent-child interaction may be obtained.
5. There is a greater likelihood of gaining helpful insights because other family members are present.

Keep in mind, however, that several cautions exist in providing assessment activity in the home. First, the assessor must be alert to the potential for a wide range of responses and interactions while in the home setting. Parents may be so comfortable that they all but ignore the assessor. Parents may assume that the "professional" has arrived to assess the child, not fully understanding that the assessment involves gaining information on the overall pattern of interaction present between the parent and the infant or toddler. Uninvolved parents, or those who show disinterest as the assessment takes place, provide the assessor with important insight on the type, quality, and frequency of parent-child interaction that takes place in the home. Although this is informative to the assessor, it may also detract from the accuracy of samples of behavior elicited during the assessment.

A second caution relates to the nature of the home environment. It may be less than optimal for elicitation of needed samples of behavior. It may be maximally distracting to the child. Hence, unreliable samples of behavior may be obtained. Attempting to assess the child while the television is on, while other children are running in and out and providing multiple opportunities for distraction, or while the parent has attention directed elsewhere for any one of a number of reasons all detract from an optimal assessment opportunity. The assessor providing services in the home environment must always keep in mind that those services are being delivered on someone else's "turf" and that there are cautions inherent in operating in a home setting.

A final comment on assessment in the home setting is that in most instances one professional completes the assessment. It is not possible to bring all members of the team into the home. Even in true transdisciplinary team models, limitations exist when only one professional provides assessment in the home. This is both a strength and a weakness, however.

CENTER-BASED ASSESSMENT

The second environment in which infant-toddler assessment activity might be provided is in a center-based delivery system. The concept of a center-based delivery system simply implies that the child is brought to the assessor in one of a variety of environments. The environments in which center-based assessment are provided are as varied as the professionals working with infants and toddlers. Infant-toddler assessment may be provided in an outpatient setting through a follow-up clinic based in a hospital. It may also be provided as part of a discharge routine in the hospital for children who have been hospitalized for a variety of medical factors. There are models in operation that provide assessment activity before discharge from the neonatal intensive care nursery, followed by outpatient evaluations on a regular basis by an early intervention team. However, the bulk of infant-toddler assessment activity is not at present provided in the medical setting.

Additional avenues of center-based assessment involve services available through community agencies designed to provide early intervention services to infants and toddlers. These may include social service agencies, private agencies, school-based assessments, university clinics, private practitioners, and outpatient rehabilitation centers. The exact makeup of the personnel involved in these environments will be varied. Regardless of the center-based environment in which infant-toddler assessment services are provided, several advantages exist. These are listed in modified form below (Filler, 1983):

1. Parents and children have greater access to staff and more services. One of the strengths of the center-based model is that additional professional expertise is usually readily available. Depending on the

model of team functioning in place, a child may be seen by an entire child assessment team or at least by one or two child assessors.
2. Parents are afforded the opportunity to interact with other parents. The benefits of this interaction should not be underestimated. It is important that parents of handicapped infants and
toddlers realize that they are not alone in their experiences. It is
quite supporting for parents to have another set of parents with
whom they might share frustrations and common experiences.
3. Should any specialized services be needed, they will be more readily available to the child.

The praciticner must likewise be aware of limitations inherent in a center-based approach to delivering infant-toddler assessment services. These
relate in large measure to the nature of the environment itself. Later chapters will point out in greater detail an overall philosophy of assessment that
involves viewing behaviors obtained on an assessment as reflecting the
child's performance on the day of the evaluation only. The assessor must
also keep in mind the threatening nature of the center, both for the child
and the parent. Unlike the home setting, in which the child is assessed in
a very familiar environment, the center-based approach requires that the
child be seen in a strange environment by persons with whom the child is
not overly familiar. This can certainly influence the samples of behavior that
are obtained during the assessment.

PROFESSIONALS INVOLVED IN
INFANT-TODDLER ASSESSMENT

One of the main points that must be recalled regarding infant-toddler assessment is that the present sytem is complex and interdependent. Many professionals are involved to varying degrees in providing
services to infants and toddlers. As a result, each potential member of
the team must become familiar with the major areas of functioning that
team members engage in. Effective interprofessional relationships, and
the degree of effectiveness that each team member displays, are facilitated by the quality of knowledge professionals have about the credentials, responsibilities, and contributions made by each team member.
Accordingly, the following information is designed to summarize the
contributions each team member brings to the overall team process
and to the delivery of infant-toddler assessment activity. The individual
professional personnel to be described include physicians, nurses, physical therapists, occupational therapists, psychologists, social workers, educators (early childhood and early childhood special education), and
speech language pathologists and audiologists. Additional disciplines may

be part of infant-toddler assessment teams; however, those indicated above constitute the bulk of disciplines represented on such teams.

PHYSICIAN

Description

Despite some arguments to the contrary, physicians are still the central figures in health care. Most people access the health care system through their physicians. This is also the case for infants and toddlers who are suspected of displaying developmental pathology. Many of these children will have factors surrounding pregnancy and delivery, or the neonatal period, that place them in a category for greater risk of displaying developmental delay. For these children in particular, entrance into systems designed to remediate developmental delay is made largely through physician referral. The issue of physician referral will be dealt with in somewhat greater detail later in this section.

   In general the medical profession is currently undergoing a significant degree of transition. Outside forces have interacted to cause physicians to alter their traditional approach toward the delivery of health care. One indication of the degree of transition taking place in medicine is that the traditional fee-for-service relationship is rapidly dying. Kamaroff (1985) points out that physicians are moving more into large group practices and networks as well as affiliating with alternative delivery systems such as health maintainance organizations (HMOs). It has been estimated that 50 percent of all physicians will be salaried employees of health systems by 1990. These changes will trickle down to the role that physicians play in the delivery of services to handicapped infants and toddlers.

   Whereas physicians have traditionally directed overall patient care, they are increasingly aware that nonphysician health care professionals also have expertise. However, the process of realizing that fact has been quite slow and protracted in many instances. To an ever-increasing degree, nonphysician health care professionals are declaring themselves as more independent than traditionally thought. This state of affairs is particularly apparent in the delivery of assessment and intervention services to handicapped infants and toddlers. Physicians are increasingly aware of a shared goal — optimal child development — that facilitates increasing cooperation between infant-toddler assessors and interventionists. Thus the overall availability and quality of services to infants and toddlers in need is enhanced. Physician referral is no longer necessary before administration of infant-toddler assessments. In fact, in many instances, a referral is made by the infant-toddler assessor to a physician following the assessment. Increased cooperation between nonphysician health care providers and physicians can do no less than significantly expand the scope and quality of services available to infants and toddlers in need.

At some point, physician services for those working with young handicapped children is essential. The greater the deviance a child displays from normal patterns of development, the greater the likelihood that the deviations are medically based. The more complex the child's medical problems, the more medical specialists the child is likely to see. Issues regarding case management arise when several medical specialties become involved. In many instances the child's pediatrician serves as case manager and liaison between medical personnel and nonphysician health care providers. Systems of this nature can be quite effective and should be emulated when appropriate.

Certification

Licensure is required in all states for medical practitioners to provide appropriate services. The attaining of a license to practice medicine depends on completion of a course of medical study from an accredited medical school. Following the course of study, an internship year is required in most instances. Many medical practitioners elect, following internship, to participate in a residency program 2 to 5 years long. The residency program provides more in-depth experience in one of a number of medical specialty areas. Medical practitioners may also elect to attain board certification in a specialty area. This involves demonstrating sufficient experience in the specialty area in which board certification is being sought as well as completing a written and oral examination. Of all the members of the health care team, physicians are subject to the most stringent certification and licensure requirements.

PHYSICAL THERAPIST

Description

The major realm of activity that physical therapists are involved in includes the planning, conducting, and evaluation of persons who display functional impairment. Physical therapists focus on individuals who present disorders related to musculoskeletal, neurologic, pulmonary, and cardiovascular systems. The goal of physical therapists is to prevent disability and pain, restore function, promote healing, and facilitate adaption to permanent disability.

Physical therapists are employed in varied settings, including hospitals (40% of physical therapists work in hospitals), home health–home care agencies, public and private schools, outpatient clinics, long-term-care facilities, academic institutions, business and industry, and private offices (the number of physical therapists involved in private practice is rapidly expanding). A growing number of physical are therapists involved primarily in providing services to pediatric populations. In such settings, the primary interest is with the child's strengths and problem areas in gross and fine motor development and sensory skills. One can readily see how these areas relate to the acquisition of normal functioning for handicapped infants and toddlers.

In most, if not all, instances the physical therapist is part of the infant-toddler assessment team. The contributions made by physical therapists to overall team functioning are significant and cannot be ignored or underestimated. The evaluation and treatment of motor disorders overlaps significantly with the child's overall development. Consequently, physical therapists interact regularly with other professionals in providing comprehensive services to infants and toddlers. Physical therapists are specifically trained to evaluate and take into consideration muscle tone, postural reactions, sensory skills, and functional motor disorders. Once deviations are detected, physical therapists are equipped to provide a course of treatment designed to alleviate the effects of motor dysfunction. In most instances the program of treatment directed toward the child with motor dysfunction is individualized to meet the child's specific needs. In addition, the physical therapist is involved to a significant degree with parents. The physical therapist may in fact design a program of treatment that the parents in large measure administer.

Certification

Certified physical therapists are qualified to provide the above-mentioned services in one of three ways. Proper credentials are gained through obtaining a bachelor's degree in physical therapy, through gaining a certificate in physical therapy after receiving a bachelor's degree in a related field, or through obtaining a graduate degree in physical therapy. Increasing numbers of physical therapists possess the graduate degree. There has been growing discussion about requiring the graduate degree as an entry-level degree to practice physical therapy. Physical therapists practice in all 50 states. Many states permit physical therapy services and evaluations without physician referral. The American Physical Therapy Association (APTA) is the national professional organization, representing approximately 45,000 physical therapists and physical therapy assistants.

OCCUPATIONAL THERAPIST

Description

Occupational therapy involves activities designed to restore, reinforce, and enhance functioning, to facilitate learning of essential skills, to reduce or correct pathologic functioning, and to promote and assist in maintaining overall health. Occupational therapy services are for the most part provided for persons whose lives have been affected by illness or injury, developmental problems, aging, or social or psychological difficulties. According to the American Occupational Therapy Association (AOTA) (1979), the activities provided by occupational therapists involve activities designed to develop, improve, or minimize debilitation and planning for and documenting the effects of such treatment.

The general scope of activities provided by occupational therapists involves the following broad areas: independent living–daily living skills, psychological and emotional daily living skills, work adaptation, sensorimotor components, sensory integration, cognitive components, psychosocial components, therapeutic adaptations, and prevention. In many instances the services provided for handicapped infants and toddlers do not distinguish between occupational therapists and physical therapists. As the child matures, services offered by occupational therapists and physical therapists may show increasing differentiation and specialization.

It is readily apparent that the scope of activities described is, in part, applicable to the types of developmental pathology observed in infants and toddlers. In actual practice a growing number of occupational therapists are concentrating the bulk of their professional activity on pediatric populations. Consequently, many occupational therapists are functioning as members of infant-toddler assessment teams. Input provided by occupational therapists on observations of developmental adequacy can be valuable for overall team activity. Input of this nature is quite helpful in planning and implementing early intervention efforts.

The AOTA represents approximately 32,000 occupational therapists and 7,500 certified occupational therapy assistants in the United States. At present occupational therapists work in hospitals, rehabilitation centers, sheltered workshops, universities, long-term-care facilities, industry, schools, home care agencies, and private practice. Approximately 20 percent of occupational therapists are independent contractors. Of those, 6 percent are engaged in private practice settings.

Certification

The minimum requirement for entry into occupational therapy includes an undergraduate degree from an accredited training program in occupational therapy. Following formal coursework a minimum of 6 months of clinical training is required as part of the training process (length of clinical training is determined by the training institution). The designation occupational therapist registered is awarded to individuals who have met these requirements and passed a national registration examination as well. The practice of occupational therapy is currently regulated in 40 jurisdictions. An increasing number of occupational therapists are pursuing advanced coursework.

SPEECH-LANGUAGE PATHOLOGIST AND AUDIOLOGIST

The speech-language pathologist and audiologist have a valuable role to play in both direct and indirect service to infants and toddlers. A growing body of evidence indicates that one of the primary areas of deficit displayed by infants of low birth weight and prematurity is that of speech and language problems. One of the most frequently mentioned areas of concern for infants and toddlers suspected of displaying developmental pathology is delayed communication development.

Speech-language pathologists and audiologists are often referred to as communication specialists. They provide services, both assessment and remedial, in a variety of settings, including public schools, colleges and universities, community speech and hearing centers, military institutions, hospitals, outpatient settings, long-term-care facilities, early intervention clinics (both center and home based), and private practice settings. The speech-language pathologist and audiologist are a valuable component of the infant-toddler assessment team.

Audiologist

The audiologist is concerned primarily with the early detection of peripheral auditory dysfunction and, when indicated, appropriate intervention. A growing number of audiologists are providing audiologic assessment before hospital discharge for infants in the intensive care nursery. Auditory brainstem response (ABR) testing is the procedure used in the intensive care nursery in many instances. The American-Speech-Language-Hearing Association (ASHA) is currently drafting guidelines regarding audiologic activity in the intensive care nursery. Regardless of when initial audiologic assessment is performed or the methods used, the infant-toddler assessment team requires accurate information on the status of the child's hearing. This is best provided by a qualified audiologist.

Speech-Language Pathologist

The speech-language pathologist is concerned with the prevention or early detection of communicative pathology. An important part of all infant-toddler assessment activity involves the determination of communicative ability. A growing body of information exists regarding the importance of prespeech experiences afforded a child and how the lack of normal prespeech opportunity affects later speech and language development. Hence speech-language pathologists are involved with children at younger and younger ages, including activity provided in the intensive care nursery. Once a child is identified as having a communicative delay, or is at risk of developing a delay, aggressive intervention services are provided. These services involve not only assessment but also the designing of treatment strategies administered by the speech-language pathologist and relying heavily on maximal parental involvement.

Certification

The minimum educational requirements for certification by ASHA include a master's degree in speech-language pathology or audiology from an accredited training program. The speech-language pathologist and the audiologist must also complete a 12-month clinical fellowship year. Both the speech-language pathologist and the audiologist must pass a national qualifying examination before being awarded the certificate of clinical competency (CCC). In addition, many states have licensure laws regulating the activity of speech-language pathologists and audiologists. There are approximately 50,000 current members of ASHA.

NURSE

Description

The nursing profession is currently undergoing significant change. This change is reflected in training, specialties, areas of nursing activity, settings of practice, and overall authority afforded nurses in various practice settings. Nurses are found in all settings in which health care services are delivered. These may include hospitals, clinics, HMOs, health departments, physician's offices, business and industry, schools, military institutions, university settings and public health care delivery systems.

Infant-toddler practitioners who work in health care settings will have regular and important contact with nursing personnel. Many teams use nursing input as a regular part of the infant-toddler assessment activity provided by the team. In some situations the nurse may function as a liaison between the team and the physician providing input to the team. The nurse can be quite valuable in interacting with parents regarding the medical aspects of intervention for those children who display developmental pathology due in large measure to medical factors.

Various specialty areas of nursing are more likely than others to be involved in infant-toddler assessment. One of these areas is rehabilitation nursing. The goal of rehabilitation nursing is to prevent complications of physical disability, restore optimal functioning, and allow the patient to adapt to an altered life-style due to the presence of a disability. Rehabilitation nursing involves both physical and social care. It is designed to assist the person and to help the family better understand and deal effectively with the presence of a disability. This can be particularly helpful in situations in which a set of parents must begin taking care of a medically fragile child for the first time in the home.

Certification

The American Nurses Association (ANA) is the professional organization for nurses. It represents approximately 200,000 members. The ANA maintains programs governing specialty certification, accredits continuing education programs, and sets standards for nursing practice, education, and credentialing. In general, the professional status of nursing has been significantly enhanced in the past decade. This is largely due to a rapid expansion in the scientific base for nursing practice as well as the increased realization that nursing has much to offer allied health care providers in both general and specific areas. Nurses today are assuming greater authority and responsibility and are more likely to hold the bachelor of science degree in nursing (BSN) or the master of science degree in nursing (MSN) from accredited nursing training programs. Following coursework, which involves both academic and clinical components, nurses are required to complete an examination before full certification. A growing number of nursing administrators also possess a doctorate degree. Licensure is required in all 50 states to practice nursing.

PSYCHOLOGIST

Description

Reviewing the manner in which psychologists are involved in providing services to infants and toddlers is quite exhaustive. Several specialty areas in psychology are involved to some degree in providing services to infants and toddlers with developmental delay. These services are directed toward both the child and the family in many instances. Some of the psychology specialty areas that the practitioner might work with include clinical, developmental, cognitive, counseling, educational, experimental, personality, psychometric-quantitative, rehabilitation, school, and social.

One byproduct of the variety of psychology specialty areas available relates to the various practice settings in which these professionals function. Psychologists are found in academic, hospital and clinical, business and government, and human service settings. In addition, a growing number of psychologists are found in private practice settings. All 50 states and the District of Columbia require an appropriate license for the independent practice of psychology.

Two psychology specialty areas that are most likely to be involved in infant-toddler assessment include the educational and developmental psychologist. The developmental psychologist is knowledgeable about general principles of how and why changes in behavior occur and what variables relate to change. The educational psychologist is most likely to be trained in educational testing and programming. Educational psychologists are often equipped to identify specific developmental problems in children and to offer appropriate suggestions for remediation. Many educational and developmental psychologists have assumed an expanded role in the early detection of developmental pathology. Hence their involvement in infant-toddler assessment activity is necessary.

The actual activities engaged in by the psychologist functioning on an infant-toddler assessment team depend more on the setting in which the activities are performed than on the psychologist's individual background. Direct time spent with parents and children will vary from setting to setting. The psychologist may assume two basic roles as a member of the team. The first is that of direct participant in the assessment activity provided and would involve interpreting assessment results. A second role that the psychologist may fulfil is as a provider of services unique to the field of psychology. These may include family intervention and adjustment, behavior management, counseling, and educational planning and intervention when so indicated. In many instances the psychologist may be in the best position to communicate team findings and recommendations to the family.

Certification

The American Psychological Association (APA) is the professional organization that has as its purpose the overall advancement of psychology as a science. The APA sets educational standards and provides input regarding certification and licensing requirements. Psychologists are regulated in part by the setting in which services are provided. For example, there are approximately 20,000 psychologists employed in public school settings. These professionals must meet certification requirements dictated by individual states, including the completion of a degree in psychology (generally a graduate degree) from an accredited training program. Psychologists who are involved in private practice must meet licensure requirements set up in each individual state. There are approximately 62,000 members in the APA, which has 42 divisions to which members may belong. The APA publishes 24 psychological journals.

SOCIAL WORKER

Description

Professionals involved in the field of social work seek to help individuals, groups, and communities reach the highest possible degree of social, mental, and psychological well-being. In general, the overall goal of social work is to reconcile the well-being of individuals with the welfare of the society in which they live. Social workers help people alter their environment as well as the ways in which they interact with family and society in general. The social worker is trained to plan for and provide services to individuals that will increase or restore their capabilities for social functioning.

There are ten primary social work specialties: (1) child welfare, (2) public welfare, (3) drug and alcohol abuse, (4) mental health, (5) health care, (6) family service, (7) developmental disabilities, (8) industry, business, and labor, (9) schools and youth, and (10) services to the aged. At present approximately one-third of social workers are found in health care settings. Social workers are usually quite active in coordinating communication between the infant-toddler assessment team and the family. As part of team functioning, depending on the particular model of team activity used, the social worker may initially interview parents and assign team members to the child based on the information received in the initial interview. Thus, the social worker is in a good position to function as the case manager for handicapped infants and toddlers.

One of the greatest contributions that social workers bring to the effective functioning of the infant-toddler assessment team is their familiarity with human development and behavior, social welfare systems and institutions, social and economic factors, and the availability of supportive services for children and their families. All members of the assessment team need background information, and this may be best obtained by the social worker. The actual activity engaged in by the social worker may vary from team to team. However, the addition of a social worker to the team is mandatory, as any professional familiar with overall team functioning can readily attest to.

Certification

The preferred academic-educational credential for social work practice is the master of social work degree (MSW). This degree includes the completion of 900 hours of supervised internship experience. Social workers are certified by the National Association of Social Workers (NASW) and licensed in 36 states. The NASW, with 90,000 members and 55 chapters, is the largest association of professional social workers in the world.

EARLY CHILDHOOD EDUCATION SPECIALIST

Description

The term *early childhood education specialist* (ECES) refers to a variety of academic disciplines that share a common interest in infants and toddlers.

Some of the specific academic disciplines that might be included under the broader meaning of ECES include (1) human growth and development, (2) child life studies, (3) developmental psychology, (4) preschool education teachers, (5) curriculum designers, and (6) persons interested in family life studies. Perhaps the best way to describe the ECES is as a professional whose major interests and skills lie in the field of applied developmental psychology with emphasis on early childhood development, early childhood education, and the relationship of these two areas to early identification of developmental pathology and subsequent early intervention (Allen, 1978).

There is a growing trend toward professional certification and specified degree requirements for those interested in early childhood education. This trend will continue and expand as current federal legislation serves to increase the scope of services available to infants and toddlers.

One distinct advantage to those who have been trained as ECES professionals is the familiarity displayed for the team concept of service delivery. In many instances the ECES has worked with a wide variety of professionals and understands the individual roles each plays as well as the collective roles played by the entire team. This can be a valuable asset to overall team activity. Although the ECES may not be involved heavily in the assessment portion of early services afforded to infants and toddlers, it is most likely that the ECES will be the professional designated to implement many of the recommendations that emanate from the team. This places the ECES in a unique position in which to view child change over time and to provide these observations to the assessment team for inclusion into follow-up evaluations.

Certification

At present all states have requirements in place that govern teacher certification. However, not all states regulate persons who provide services to infants and toddlers, especially if such services are provided outside the public school setting. Thus, many professionals providing services to infants and toddlers (early intervention services) are not governed by licensing or certification regulations. This is due in part to the fact that most states do not currently mandate the provision of services to infants and toddlers; hence, there is no need to regulate practitioners who provide such services. In those settings in which state or federal dollars are the primary source of funding, some requirements for provider expertise are in effect.

MODELS FOR EARLY CASEFINDING

Infant-toddler assessment should be conducted in the context of a philosophical viewpoint consistent with a clear understanding of the efficacy of early intervention. That is, the infant-toddler assessor should be convinced of the benefits of early detection and treatment of developmental pathology.

In essence, discussing the benefits of early casefinding is identical to discussing the benefits of early intervention. Early detection and early intervention should not be viewed as separate activities but as one and the same. Thus, early identification should lead to early intervention. These activities are linked in a manner that suggests that early casefinding is a wasted activity apart from early intervention. Realizing the importance of early identification and intervention leads to a discussion of the most effective manner of detecting developmental delay at the earliest possible age.

The provision of services to infants and toddlers displaying developmental pathology is a thoroughly defensible notion. Common sense and empirical evidence (see Chapter 1) dictate that attention be given to children at the earliest possible age to sustain their development and ensure optimal growth. Without special, comprehensive intervention, children with known disability and those at risk for developing such problems may not achieve optimal levels of developmental skill acquisition. The aim of early intervention is to prevent disorders that may arise from various biologic or environmental factors. Despite evidence to the contrary, many children are not referred for intervention services at the earliest ages. The prevailing attitude in these instances is "wait and see" and "perhaps the child will outgrow the problem." Soboloff (1979) has stated quite well the need for early detection of developmental pathology, saying that "it can no longer be accepted that treatment does not begin until the child is three years of age" (p. 424). It might be added that it makes little sense not to direct attention toward early detection of developmental pathology.

In a study designed to assess how early children with developmental pathology were detected, Palfrey, Singer, Walker, and Butler (1987) studied five metropolitan communities. Parent-interview data were collected on 1,726 children regarding how early the child's problem was detected. For the conditions studied, the range for age at identification was quite large. Four percent of the children were identified at birth, 16.4 percent before age 3 years, and 28.7 percent before age 5 years. The period from 5 to 7 years was the most active for identification of problems, with 47.9 percent diagnosed during the early elementary years. The special needs of the remaining 23.3 percent of the children were detected at age 8 years or older.

Part of the range present in these results is due to the widely divergent nature of the primary handicaps that were included as definitions of developmental pathology. However, the fact that more than 50 percent of handicaps were detected after age 5 lends strong support to the fact that many children are not detected as displaying developmental pathology at the optimal ages. In these cases early intervention is not probable, since the disorder is not detected until later (age 5 years and above).

It is clear from these results that much must be done to arrive at a more effective manner of sharing responsibilities for the early detection of developmental pathology. This responsibility must be shared by medical and allied health professionals alike. The need for shared responsibility in early detection of delay is amplified by additional findings in the Palfrey, Singer, Walker, and Butler (1987) study. These findings indicate that low-prevalence disabilities are far more likely to be identified by a physician than by someone else, although nonphysicians did identify 25 percent of the mentally retarded children and 36 percent of the hearing impaired children. By contrast, the high-prevalence disabilities were more likely to be identified by someone other than a physician, most commonly a teacher or other school professional. Physicians diagnosed only 44 percent of the hyperactive children and less than 25 percent of speech impairments, emotional problems, learning disabilities, and other developmental problems.

Any model for the detection of developmental pathology at an early age must have in mind various target populations at risk of displaying developmental delay. Chapter 2 outlines in some detail categories of children at known risk. An additional paradigm of viewing those children who will require assessment early in life is presented by Tjossem (1976), who describes three categories of vulnerable infants.

1. *Established risk.* Babies with established risk are defined as those "whose early appearing aberrant development is related to medical disorders of known etiology bearing well known expectancies for developmental outcome within specific ranges of developmental delay" (p. 5). The child with Down syndrome is an example of a child in this category.

2. *Environmental risk.* Children at environmental risk are "biologically sound infants for whom life experiences including maternal and family care, health care, opportunities for expression of adaptive behaviors, and patterns of physical and social stimulation are sufficiently limiting to the extent that, without corrective intervention, they impart high probability for delayed development" (p. 5).

3. *Biologic risk.* Those at biologic risk are defined by Tjossem (1976) as "infants presenting a history of prenatal, perinatal, neonatal, and early developmental events suggestive of biological insults to the developing central nervous system and which, either singly or collectively, increases the probability of later appearing aberrant development" (p. 5).

It is precisely the categories of children described in Chapter 2 and by Tjossem who need service delivery systems that effectively monitor developmental progress and provide appropriate intervention in the presence of aberrant development.

MODEL SYSTEMS

IOWA

Since 1978 the state of Iowa has had in operation a statewide system for the screening, tracking, and referral of high-risk infants. The system was put into effect in response to a large body of data indicating that comprehensive care is especially important for children who are at risk for, or who already have, disabling conditions because the earlier disabilities are detected and treated, the greater the chance for remediation and the smaller the impact of these disabilities on children, families, and society (Blackman and Hein, 1985). Funding for the system has come from the state, Crippled Children's Services, and federal and private grants. The goal of the program is to provide statewide services accessible to all eligible children. Eligibility is determined by a set of entry criteria (Table 3-2).

Infants with readily detectable conditions at birth are not enrolled in the program but are referred immediately for appropriate educational or therapeutic services. Actual screening and evaluation services are provided by pediatric nurse practitioners (PNPs) in seven sites around the state. The children are screened by PNPs at 4, 9, 18, and 30 months of age. The screening involves the administration of a standard infant screening instrument (Denver Developmental Screening Test) and a physical examination provided by a physician. Based on the screening assessment results, the child may be referred for further services. These may include services available in school or private settings and be either home or center based. One

TABLE 3-2. Eligibility criteria for the high-risk follow-up program

1. Birth weight < 1,500 gm
2. Respiratory distress syndrome
3. Other forms of respiratory distress that require mechanical ventilation for 2 hours or more
4. Bacterial meningitis as well as all forms of central nervous system infection
5. Asphyxia neonatorum, as indicated by a 5-minute Apgar score of < 7
6. Hypoglycemia
7. Neonatal seizures
8. Hypotonia at the discharge examination
9. Other infants who are felt to be at risk by physician such as infants who were small for date or those entering environments that present severe psychosocial concerns

Source: Adapted from J. Blackman and H. Hein (1985). Iowa's system for screening and tracking high risk infants. *American Journal of Diseases of Children, 139,* 826.

very positive benefit of this system is that 75 percent of all infants who ultimately did display aberrant patterns of development were identified by 15 months of age. These results differ markedly from those reported in the Palfrey, Singer, Walker, and Butler (1987) study cited previously.

MASSACHUSETTS

Massachusetts has a state mandate for early intervention that requires the state health department to provide, facilitate, and coordinate services to handicapped and at-risk infants from birth to 3 years of age. The Massachusetts law does not specify what services must be provided other than to stipulate that a team approach must be used. The team is defined as a developmental educator and two others. Regardless of professional discipline, Massachusetts' early intervention services must be family centered, team oriented, and related to developmental outcomes.

NEW JERSEY

Similar to Massachusetts is the program in place in New Jersey. Services are provided to qualified children from birth. In New Jersey an interdepartmental committee has developed approval criteria for any public or private agency to receive funding for services under the state's early intervention program. The services are provided by a team that must be composed of appropriately credentialed professionals, including ECESs, speech-language pathologists, occupational therapists, or physical therapists. In addition, at least two of the following are required: psychologist, registered nurse, and social worker. Other specialists are permitted as needed. Most referrals in New Jersey to the early intervention program come from physicians in the private sector.

MARYLAND

In Maryland, early childhood programs are defined as those programs designed to provide intervention directly to handicapped children from birth through 4 years. The services provided are directed toward the child, the parents, or both. The Maryland Department of Education regulations define the services provided as including physical and occupational therapy, speech pathology and audiology, psychological services, recreation, counseling services, and medical services for diagnostic and evaluation purposes. In Maryland, state and local education agencies coordinate with state and local health departments and the University Affiliated Faculty in Baltimore on an ad hoc basis to provide health-related services.

TEXAS

A comprehensive early identification and intervention program was initiated in Texas in 1981. Known as the Early Childhood Intervention Program (ECI), its purpose is to identify and provide needed services to children from birth to age 6 who are or appear to be at risk of developmental delay.

The components of ECI in Texas include (1) an advisory committee, made up of 15 members who provide advice on service delivery issues; (2) a public awareness and training program, which educates the public about the importance of early detection of developmental delay; (3) monitoring and evaluation, to ensure that all rules and regulations are adhered to; (4) centralized tracking and follow-up, to keep records; (5) service delivery, to provide services in areas in the state in which none currently exists; and (6) a grant review process, which selects programs for funding through a competitive process of review. An individualized approach is used for each child.

The three major sources of referrals to ECI in Texas are physicians, hospitals, and parents. When a child is referred to ECI, he or she is screened by a team of professionals from various disciplines who then meet with the parents to discuss developmental and educational needs. The actual services provided include educational, medical, speech and hearing, physical therapy, occupational therapy, parent training, diagnostic medical evaluations, diagnostic social evaluations, day care, respite care, case management, and parent information and education. The bulk of children served through ECI in Texas are in the 13 to 36 month range.

A variety of measures have been taken to gauge the effectiveness of ECI activities. Overall, the services provided have been shown to be quite effective in helping children achieve optimal developmental performance.

*   *   *

Other programs have been in operation for varying amounts of time in different parts of the United States. For the most part, these other programs are primarily local and likely not part of statewide comprehensive activity. The examples cited above represent activity, sufficiently funded, to meet the early identification needs of entire states.

SUMMARY

Large strides have been taken in recent years to put into place effective systems designed to detect developmental pathology at early ages. In addition, a variety of strategies have been used and tested to make the actual delivery of assessment and intervention services as effective as possible. Team management issues, professional discipline issues, assessment settings, service delivery models, parent involvement, and interdisciplinary issues have been explored. In one sense the attention that has been directed toward these issues has culminated, at least in part, in the passage of powerful federal legislation designed to make the provision of services to handicapped infants and toddlers accessible to all. Rather than viewing the passage of this legislation as the achievement of a goal, it should be viewed as the opening of a door. This door represents a unique opportunity to provide a spectrum of services to those most vulnerable in our society — infants and toddlers who are developmentally delayed.

Palfrey, Singer, Walker, and Butler (1987) indicate that early identification of developmental pathology involves three components: the natural history of childhood disorders, the techniques of screening and diagnosis, and the delivery systems available for applying these techniques. Many handicapped conditions are being detected very early, but the rate of early diagnosis for various other disorders is not as high as it should be. The low rate of early identification for speech disorders, hyperactivity, learning disorders, and other developmental problems is unacceptable. Strategies to detect the presence of these disorders before school age, and earlier, must be refined and expanded. An assertive approach by medical and all health care professionals for early identification and intervention must be stressed. Enhanced coordination between primary care physicians and other child development specialists must result. When problems are detected, physicians and all health care professionals should have a readily available referral source for further elucidation of the problem and a clear working relationship with agencies, private and public, so that services can be promptly provided. The detection of developmental pathology before 1 year of age should be a major goal of developmental specialists. These issues present significant challenges to the health care system. These challenges can best be regarded as interdisciplinary, requiring cooperation from all team members to pursue them jointly and effectively.

STUDY QUESTIONS

1. Describe in your own words the team concept.
2. What are the three team functioning models described in this chapter? What do you see as the strengths and weaknesses of each?
3. What are the various settings in which infant-toddler assessment may take place? What must the assessor keep in mind when considering each of these settings?

4. What professionals might constitute the typical assessment team? What are the roles and functions of each team member?
5. Describe in your own words what you see as the "model" program of early casefinding and infant-toddler assessment.

REFERENCES

Allen, K. (1978). The early childhood specialist. In K. Allen (Ed.), *Early intervention: A team approach*. Austin, TX: PRO-ED.

American Occupational Therapy Association. (1979). *Uniform terminology for reporting occupational therapy services*. Rockville, MD: Author.

Blackman, J., & Hein, H. (1985). Iowa's system for screening and tracking high risk infants. *American Journal of Diseases of Children, 139*, 826.

Blayney, K. (1986). Restructuring the health care labor force: The rise of the multi-skilled health practitioner. *Alabama Journal of Medical Science, 23*, 277.

Briggs, M. (1989). Interdisciplinary team: Goals and strategies. Paper presented at the Infants and Toddlers Communication and Intervention Workshop, Bethesda, MD

Cornett, B., & Chabon, S. (1988). The clinical practice of speech-language pathology. Columbus: Merrill.

Filler, J. (1983). Service models for handicapped infants. In G. Garwood and R. Fewell (Eds.), *Educating handicapped infants*. Rockville, MD: Aspen Publications.

Holm, V. & McCartin, R. (1978). Interdisciplinary child development team: Team issues and training in interdisciplinariness. In K. Allen (Ed.), *Early intervention: A team approach*. Austin, TX: PRO-ED.

Kamaroff, A. (1985). Quality assurance in 1985. *Medical Care, 23*, 277.

Kile, J., & Rossetti, L. (1988, November). Neurodevelopmental and audiologic assessment of infants and toddlers. Short course presented at the Annual Convention of the American Speech-Language-Hearing Association. Boston.

Lowe, J., & Herranen, M. (1978). Conflict in teamwork: Understanding roles and relationships. *Social Work in Health Care, 3*, 323.

McCormick, L., & Lee, C. (1979). Public law 94-142: Mandated partnerships. *American Journal of Occupational Therapy, 33*, 586.

Melvin, J. (1980). Interdisciplinary and multidisciplinary activities and the American Congress of Rehabilitation Medicine. *Archives of Physical Medicine and Rehabilitation, 61*, 379.

Palfrey, J., Singer, J., Walker, D., & Butler, J. (1987). Early identification of children's special needs: A study of five metropolitan communities. *Journal of Pediatrics, 3*, 651.

Pellegrino, E. (1977). The allied health professions: The problems and potentials for maturity. *Journal of Allied Health, 6*, 25–29.

Rossetti, L. (1986). *High risk infants: Identification, assessment, and intervention*. Austin, TX: PRO-ED.

Soboloff, H. (1979). Developmental enrichment programs. *Developmental Medicine and Child Neurology, 21*, 423.

Sutherland-Cornett, B., & Chabon, S. (1988). *The clinical practice of speech-language pathology*. Columbus, OH: Merrill Publishing Company.

Tjossem, T. (1976). *Intervention strategies for high risk infants and young children*. Baltimore: University Park Press.

Watkins, R. (1983). Medical rehabilitation in the present and a promise for the future. *Annals of the Academy of Medicine, 12*, 438.

CHAPTER   4

General and Specific Assessment Considerations

General Assessment
Considerations
   Why Assess Infants and
      Toddlers?
   Assessment Defined
   The Predictive Ability of Tests
      of Infant-Toddler
      Development
   Viewing Assessment Results

Specific Assessment
Considerations
   Correcting for Prematurity
   Significance of Catch-Up
      Growth
   Need for Serial Assessment
   When to Initiate Assessment
      Activity
   Assessment Intervals
   Determination of Infant State
   Assessing Atypical Infants and
      Toddlers

   Summary

   Study Questions

   References

The conclusion of Chapter 3 presented a variety of challenges facing the infant-toddler specialist. Certainly not the least of these is the gaining of information by the skilled assessor from which judgments about developmental adequacy can be made. It is precisely this information that serves as the basis for a number of decisions regarding early intervention. The implications of gaining valid assessment data are quite wide.

Perhaps the best manner in which to underscore the importance of infant-toddler assessment is to point out the wide applications of assessment data for an increasing array of persons. Parents are interested in accurate assessment data since important decisions concerning child placement, various medical factors, and measures of progress are based on accurate results. Researchers require valid assessment results to develop new and innovative strategies to detect developmental pathology at the earliest possible age. Early childhood educators require reliable assessment data, since both program and curriculum decisions rest in part on the effectiveness of various program models and curricula employed. Physicians rely on assessment data for assistance in monitoring overall developmental progress and for viewing medically oriented interventions in light of their impact on later developmental performance. Legislators and other policymakers require reliable assessment information as legislative and program delivery decisions are made and as existing programs are refined to increase the effectiveness of early intervention services.

Perhaps the group in greatest need of accurate assessment data is the infants and toddlers who require early intervention services. As early childhood practitioners will attest, infant-toddler intervention begins at least in part with a complete and thorough understanding of the present level of developmental skill mastery a child exhibits. Where to start in intervention, changes in both the infant or toddler and the family, and the overall effectiveness of the intervention provided can best be demonstrated through the collection of dependable, reliable, and accurate assessment data. The importance of accuracy in assessment is clearly established when viewed in light of those who benefit from it.

GENERAL ASSESSMENT CONSIDERATIONS

WHY ASSESS INFANTS AND TODDLERS?

Infant-toddler assessors should operate from a theoretical framework that assists them in understanding why infant-toddler assessment is so important. Knowing who is interested in accurate assessment results is only one way of elaborating on the importance of infant-toddler assessment. As the process of infant-toddler assessment is considered, several additional reasons that lend importance to the process emerge. The following discussion attempts to answer the question, "Why assess infants and toddlers?"

Early Detection of Developmental Pathology

Early intervention for infants and toddlers with developmental delay or for those at risk of displaying developmental delay is no longer an option. Legislation described in Chapter 1 elaborates on the mandate to find and intervene for children who are vulnerable to developmental pathology and the accompanying educational and social consequences of such delay. A large body of literature clearly demonstrates the importance of early detection of developmental delay. The process begins, in large measure, with early detection and assessment. Hence, one of the primary purposes of infant-toddler assessment is the early detection of developmental pathology. Early detection may use risk registry information regarding potential for later developmental sequelae, depend on the developmental screening afforded all infants on leaving the intensive care nursery, or the screening performed as part of well-baby evaluations. Whatever the strategy employed, either formal through norm-referenced assessment instruments or informal through the use of child development checklists, the overall purpose is the same — to identify, as early as possible, children who display developmental pathology regardless of cause or degree.

In many instances, early identification and intervention for children with a developmental delay can prevent the subsequent manifestation of serious secondary problems and may significantly reduce the impact of the overall developmental delay noted. Appropriate referrals to needed professionals can be made, and early intervention services can be initiated. The benefits of early detection are substantial, not the least of which is the long-term cost effectiveness of detecting children in need of special educational opportunities early and providing such opportunities. One of the major purposes of infant-toddler assessment is thus to find children requiring early intervention services as soon as possible.

Decide on Appropriate Intervention

Following initial screening and assessment, a decision must be made regarding the child's need for appropriate early intervention services. The decision might include the need for overall developmental enrichment activities or for intervention targeting a specific skill area such as communication or motor skills. Assessment activity, depending on the exact nature of the assessment performed, might indicate that a center- versus a home-based approach would be most successful. The results of the assessment may reveal specific skill areas that should be focused on as areas of strength. It may be possible to determine specific curricula that would be most appropriate for a particular child. Some assessment instruments are helpful in providing the early interventionist with direction regarding the specific direction early intervention activity should take. However, no instruments exist that specifically direct intervention regarding frequency, target behaviors, and duration of intervention efforts. Because intervention involves the caregivers, assessment must include some information regarding the caregivers' adequacy to assist in the overall intervention effort. All intervention efforts are enhanced when reliable assessment data are readily available.

Monitor Child and Family Change

Previous discussions regarding the nature and significance of etiologic factors pointed out that rarely does the child or the family remain the same over time. A transactional relationship exists between the two. The child's status affects the family; likewise, a host of family factors affect the child. Thus, one of the main benefits of assessment is the ability to monitor and gauge child-family change. Several specific instruments designed to assist in monitoring family change will be outlined in Chapter 6. These instruments allow the assessor to measure and monitor objectively the degree to which the family is meeting the child's unique needs and the degree to which the intervention being provided is meeting the family's identified needs. Data of this nature provide the assessor with important information that can be considered when making short- and long-term decisions regarding the family-focus aspects of intervention.

Child change issues relate to other possible problems that are secondary to the initial reason for concern. In addition, totally new areas of concern may become evident. These can only be detected as assessment, over time, is undertaken. The need for regular assessment is obvious and will be discussed in greater detail later in this chapter. One fact remains consistent as practitioners provide a variety of early intervention and assessment services: Children and families experience change, and as that change occurs it must be monitored to allow the infant-toddler practitioner to intervene effectively when appropriate. These changes may relate to new areas of concern as well as to areas of family strength that must be used to provide a comprehensive and effective intervention program for infants and toddlers.

Monitor Program Effectiveness

Another significant factor that must be considered when determining why infant-toddler assessment is necessary relates to monitoring the effectiveness of intervention services provided. The efficacy of early intervention has not been investigated as systematically as is needed, but there will be more studies as more infants and toddlers receive services.

One definite measure of the efficacy of early intervention programs is the degree of developmental progress observed in the children served. This type of child change is best measured through the use of norm-referenced assessment instruments. Whether the instruments used to monitor child change are global or domain specific, these measures do give important insight into the effectiveness of the intervention services being provided.

Child change measures are by no means the only manner in which to view program effectiveness. However, if the infants and toddlers receiving intervention services demonstrate significant progress as a result of the activities provided, then one may assume that the treatment is efficacious. In instances where specific family-oriented goals have been set with an individualized family services plan (IFSP), the meeting of these goals is an important indicator of program effectiveness. Some of the instruments outlined in Chapter 6 are helpful in meeting this purpose.

Overall, evaluation of early intervention programs has generally focused on measuring child change. A few programs (and assessment instruments) have measured training impact on parents and caregivers; even fewer have collected information on other relevant variables, such as change in attitude, cost factors, or longitudinal effects. Assessment and evaluation should determine the format and success of early intervention for individual children as well as the impact of programs on groups of children. Assessment provides guidance for the development of individual and family intervention plans, feedback about the success of individual programming for children and families, and a means for determining the value of an intervention program for groups or subgroups of program participants.

Predictive Purposes

An additional factor that surfaces when considering the purposes of infant-toddler assessment relates to predicting long-term developmental expectations for children who display developmental pathology, or those at risk of doing so. Information presented in Chapter 2 describes various categories of children who are known to display, or who are at significant risk of displaying, developmental delay. In short, the infant-toddler assessor will be involved in assessment activity with those infants and toddlers who display unusual rates of development, those with known developmental disorders, deficits, or disabilities, those with hidden handicaps, and those with increased risk of displaying pathologic patterns of development due to biologic or environmental factors.

The ability to predict ultimate developmental outcome for any individual child within these categories would be of significant help to a wide range of persons. However, this ability does not exist. As a result, the infant-toddler assessor is not able to predict long-term developmental expectations for the vast majority of children who will be seen. This is particularly true if the assessor attempts to predict future expectations based on a single assessment opportunity. Impressions can be formed regarding future recommendations, but the assessor must be willing at all times to modify these initial impressions as a result of additional assessment opportunities or new information. Hence, prediction is a tenuous enterprise and should be avoided as much as possible. A more complete discussion of the problems inherent in viewing the results of infant-toddler assessment in a predictive manner is discussed later in this chapter.

ASSESSMENT DEFINED

Although the term *assessment* may have various meanings to infant-toddler practitioners, assessment as presented in this text is defined as any activity either formal (through the use of norm-referenced criteria) or informal (through the use of developmental profiles or checklists, including information gained from a variety of sources) that is designed to elicit accurate and reliable infant behaviors (or information) on which developmental skill status may be inferred (Rossetti, 1986). In essence, assessment is a paradigm for data collection. After collecting the necessary data in one of several ways, the assessor is responsible for attaching the proper significance to the samples of behavior obtained. Assessment as a data-collection tool can be broken into six potential strategies for the collection of necessary data. Each of these will be discussed below.

Formal Observations

Formal observation can be described as any observational opportunities in which the assessor follows a prescribed format in looking for specific examples of developmental performance. Observations of this nature may be made without the child's awareness that such observations are occurring. The assessor may view a child at play or interacting with caregivers to determine if appropriate patterns of environmental interaction exist. The examiner knows more or less what he or she is looking for and makes inferences regarding overall skill mastery based on the samples of behavior observed. Formal observational opportunities may take place in the home or in a more formal setting, such as a school or clinic.

Informal Observations

Informal observations are made by the examiner in a less formal and more spontaneous manner. The astute assessor realizes that in a very real sense, infant-toddler assessment begins at the moment the examiner lays eyes on the child. How many times has the experienced examiner noted that the child displayed a particular behavior while the parent was being interviewed but that same behavior could not be elicited during formal test administration? Observations such as this are quite valuable to the assessor, and one must be alert to the child's informally demonstrating behavior that may not be present in more formal settings. Informal observations may be made in any setting, but these types of opportunities may be most readily available in the home.

Direct Testing

Direct testing involves administering an established assessment instrument designed to yield objective data that can be translated into a more objective description of developmental skill mastery. Descriptions obtained through the administration of formal tests may include age equivalency scores, global skill mastery scores, skill attainment indexes in specific developmental domains, developmental quotients, percentile ranks for global and skill-specific performance, and intelligence quotient (IQ) scores. Direct testing is more formal and is usually performed in a clinical, school, or hospital setting.

There are advantages and disadvantages to direct testing. One disadvantage is that the behaviors that are acceptable for the passage of a particular item on a test are narrowly defined, and a child may demonstrate behaviors that are similar but that do not meet the specific criteria indicated in test administration instructions. An advantage is that objective data are yielded that simplify later comparisons for evaluative purposes for child change measures as well as for program effectiveness measures.

Parental Report

Parents have shown themselves to be a valuable source of information about their children's behavior. Although the parents may not have a strong ability to interpret the significance of various behaviors, the information they provide can be used by examiners in making judgments on skill mastery for a particular child.

In an attempt to clarify the reliability of data provided by parents, McCormick, Shapiro, and Starfield (1982) examined factors associated with maternal opinions of infant development. Parent interviews and child observations were performed on 4,783 children age 1 year. The majority (87%, or 4,161) of infants in the study were considered by their mothers to be developing normally for their age. Of those 622 children who were considered by their mothers as developing slowly, nearly 70 percent (435) were actually within normal range based on direct observation of child performance. Maternal opinions of slow development reflected infant health status (birth weight), hospitalization, congenital anomalies, and use of physician services. Social factors such as low maternal education and sex of the child also influenced maternal opinions regarding development. Coplan (1982) likewise examined parental accuracy in estimating the developmental performance of their children and reported that parents' descriptions of their children's behavior were usually accurate, even though their interpretations frequently were not. Results such as these reveal that there is some assurance that data provided by parents can be counted on to give a fairly accurate picture of the child's behavioral capabilities.

Teacher Report

Information provided by teachers or early childhood educators can be a valuable source of accurate and reliable data on infant-toddler behavior. It may be possible in some instances for the early childhood educator to accompany the parents as the assessor initiates assessment activity. It may also be possible for the assessor to observe the child in the classroom or the home as the teacher administers a program of early intervention. In some instances the early childhood education specialist provides both assessment and educational services. In such instances the assessor-teacher is able to use behaviors observed as part of the program of early intervention as well as behaviors gained during formal assessment. Teacher reports include important observations related to child change as a child progresses through intervention efforts. The presence of developmental progress as a direct result of intervention can be of value to the assessor. Likewise, if a child makes little or no progress during intervention activity, the assessor can use that information in putting together a more complete understanding of the child's overall developmental level and future expectations. Data obtained from the teacher report must not be overlooked if a full understanding of infant-toddler behaviors is desired.

Medical Personnel Reports

Medical records can be an important source of data for the infant-toddler assessor. Hospital discharge summaries, reports generated while the child sees any one of a number of potential medical specialists, and data gained from the results of routine medical followup can be very beneficial to the assessor. For those children who exhibit one or more high risk factors (low birth weight, prematurity, and associated medical complications), knowledge of medical history can certainly assist the assessor in better understanding the samples of behavior observed regardless of the data-collection technique used.

Children who present a history of serious medical complications, or who report ongoing medical problems, have a greater likelihood of displaying continued patterns of developmental pathology. The assessor must be aware of the child's medical history, particularly the health history, for the months before the actual assessment. The experienced assessor highly values data gained from medical records. Access to medical records may be difficult depending on the setting in which the assessment activity is performed. For the assessor functioning in a hospital setting, information should be readily available. Medical records can be requested from appropriate personnel regardless of the setting in which the assessment takes place. In addition, parents or caregivers should be able to provide basic information regarding a particular child's medical history and background.

In addition to access to medical information, the assessor should be familiar with the potential longitudinal effects of various medical complications experienced by children who fit high-risk or known developmental delay–mental retardation categories. Chapter 2 provides a basic description of several factors that contribute to developmental pathology and that should be understood by the infant-toddler assessor. The increased need for additional hospitalization for various reasons for certain categories of children makes adequate environmental exposure more difficult, thus affecting developmental change (see Table 2–8).

THE PREDICTIVE ABILITY OF TESTS
OF INFANT-TODDLER DEVELOPMENT

The usefulness of infant tests as predictors of subsequent development has been the subject of much debate, ranging from assertions of the tests' uselessness to cautious optimism concerning their value. Thus, there is still considerable controversy over whether developmental tests during the infant-toddler years have predictive value. It is imperative that the infant-toddler assessor have a clear understanding of this issue. Unawareness of the inherent limitations in trying to make long-term predictions based on early test results will serve to frustrate both the assessor and the parents.

A review of existing literature on the predictive ability of tests of infant development for healthy infants and toddlers reveals that available tests have not fared well. Hence, the supposition that measured developmental ability at one point should be closely related to measured developmental ability at a later point is not a sound one for healthy infants and toddlers. The situation is clearly more complicated in the case of a child who is displaying a developmental delay or for one who is at risk of displaying such a delay due to biologic or environmental factors. Although present knowledge of normal infant development does support the presence of a developmental sequence that leads to increased skill mastery, knowledge of the relationship between certain aspects of skill learning and other developmental performance areas is still limited. Thus, it is possible that a child at a young age will display a delay in a particular area that may have only minimal impact on other parameters of development.

Zelazo, Zelazo, and Kolb (1972) point out at least three major considerations on assessment that are important to keep in mind during the infant-toddler years: (1) brain damage can be extensive and severe without necessarily impairing cognitive ability; (2) environmental factors can significantly affect intellectual development in a negative way; and (3) a complete understanding of the specific test items is not available. The fact that environmental factors can negatively impact intellectual development has been supported by several additional investigators (Escalona, 1982; McCall, Hogarty, and Hurlbut, 1972; Siegel, 1981).

In general a variety of factors influence the predictive ability of tests administered in infancy and childhood. These include social factors, medical factors, whether the child has received any degree of infant-toddler intervention, the age at which the child was assessed, the amount and type of stimulation afforded the child in the home, and parental expectations based on the presence of medical complications that the child may have experienced early in life.

VIEWING ASSESSMENT RESULTS

The infant-toddler assessor must choose the manner in which to view and use results obtained from assessment activity. Although other options exist, either a predictive or a prescriptive approach may be used for organizing assessment results. The previous discussion of the tenuous nature of viewing assessment outcomes should alert the assessor to the limitations inherent in viewing results in a predictive manner.

Prescriptive View of Assessment Results

In the prescriptive approach, results are interpreted in an attempt to understand better the nature of the suspected delay to decide on programming, to determine specific etiology, or simply to answer the question, "What is the next step of action based on the assessment results just obtained?"

Various outcomes are possible when results are viewed in a prescriptive manner. It may be that a specific etiology is suspected, and thus efforts to prevent future occurrences of a similar event can be initiated. In answering the "What next?" question, it may be determined that other members of the interdisciplinary team are needed in varying degrees to assist in providing a comprehensive strategy for intervention. It may also be determined that further medical intervention is necessary to reduce secondary concerns that arise. The "What next?" question may likewise indicate that the parents need genetic counseling. The results of the assessment may provide information regarding intervention recommendations, both in specific skill areas to target for intervention and in specific curriculum or strategy for intervention activity. Assessment results may also indicate how frequently the child should be seen for reevaluation. Catch-up growth can be monitored and important data collected regarding child change. All these possibilities spring from viewing assessment results in a manner that allows new information about how to meet each infant's or toddler's needs to be included.

SPECIFIC ASSESSMENT CONSIDERATIONS

CORRECTING FOR PREMATURITY

A basic premise on which infant-toddler assessment is founded is that an individual child's performance is considered appropriate or not compared with the expected performance of children of similar age. Each time the assessor initiates assessment activity, no matter what form that activity ultimately takes, the assessor is attempting to answer the question, "Is this child doing what should be expected of a child of similar age?" If the child is displaying age-appropriate performance overall, then it is expected that a normal sequence of developmental skill mastery is in operation, and no specific recommendations are needed. However, if assessment results indicate that developmental skill mastery is not consistent with what should be expected of children of similar age, then the assessor must ask, "What next?" Samples of performance obtained on assessment results may be compared across developmental domains or may be specific to a particular developmental domain.

Chapter 2 presented information regarding the increased incidence of developmental pathology in children of low birth weight and prematurity. As a result, a unique set of circumstances exists for the assessor when he or she expects to obtain reliable assessment data on populations of children with a history of prematurity. As the survival rate increases for low birthweight and premature children, important questions arise on what constitutes the measuring stick to compare these infants and toddlers with.

The specific question that faces the assessor when activity is directed toward infants and toddlers who were born prematurely is whether to calculate the child's age based on the date of birth (chronologic age) or correct the chronologic age for the degree of prematurity (corrected age). A secondary issue relates to the age at which correction for prematurity should cease and the child should be compared with chronologic-age peers in an attempt to determine developmental adequacy.

For example, a child who is born 2 months early (32 weeks gestational age instead of the normal 40 weeks) can be considered a 4-month-old or a 2-month-old child when assessed four months after birth. This is a particularly important consideration because developmental adequacy or inadequacy following the administration of a particular infant-toddler test depends on which age is used.

The discussion of correction for prematurity is related to a broader discussion of what the infant has lost when deprived of normal in utero experiences due to premature delivery. A significant degree of physical and neurologic growth is known to take place in the last trimester of in utero development (Hunt, 1981; Siegel, 1983). Infants born prematurely are deprived of these important weeks, and the comparison of their development with that of full-term infants has been suggested as inappropriate. As a result, it has typically been the practice to correct for the degree of prematurity during the first 2 years of life (Hunt, 1981).

Siegel (1983) studied the consequences of correcting developmental test scores for degree of prematurity in matched groups of full-term and pre-term children. The children were administered a series of developmental tests at various ages (4, 8, 12, 18, and 24 months). At each point (age of test administration) the uncorrected scores of the pre-term children were significantly lower than those of the full-term children. However, corrected scores for the pre-term children during their first year of life were more highly correlated with test scores at 3 and 5 years. Thus, subtracting the degree of prematurity (weeks) from chronologic age expectations for infants less than 1 year of age appeared to be a more accurate predictor and better reflected later developmental performance.

Further analysis of the data revealed that from 12 months on, the uncorrected scores also displayed a high correlation with test performance at 3 and 5 years of age. In other words, correcting for prematurity, and using the corrected score in judgments about developmental adequacy, appeared to be a more appropriate manner for viewing infant test results, particularly for children less than 12 months of age. After 12 months of age both scores (corrected and uncorrected) had high correlations with later developmental performance. The author concluded by stating that "the use of correction for degree of prematurity may be appropriate in the early months, but after one year of age, there were no significant differences between predictive ability of the corrected and uncorrected scores" (p. 1187). The above results reflect a change of opinion expressed by Siegel, who in 1979 indicated that correction for prematurity was not necessary (Siegel, 1979).

Other investigators are concerned about overcorrection for prematurity. Miller, Dubowitz, and Palmer (1984) investigated whether correcting for prematurity was of help when using later developmental assessment instruments. In the Miller study, 114 preterm infants were asessed at 6, 9, 12, and 18 months. Uncorrected developmental quotients identified 76 percent of the children who showed neurologic abnormalities at 1 year of age. The abnormalities detected included dystonia, cerebral palsy, and motor delays.

Corrected developmental quotients identified only 11 percent of such children. The authors concluded that overcorrection took place and contributed to misleading interpretations of assessment results.

Similar results were obtained by Hunt and Rhodes (1977) and by Elliman, Bryan, Elliman, and Dubowitz (1985). Hunt and Rhodes followed the cognitive development of preterm infants during the first year of life. The Bayley Scale of Infant Development was administered to 56 infants divided into four groups based on gestational age. Results revealed that corrected age scores from 3 to 12 months were six to seven points above those of the full-term control group of infants. Thus it appeared that adjusted scores, based on degree of prematurity, were overcorrecting. The Elliman study followed a cohort of 198 preterm children during the first 3 years of life. The results of the Denver Developmental Screening Test (DDST) and the Griffiths Mental Development Scale (GMDS) were compared. Results indicated that overcorrection for prematurity did take place, as evidenced by higher numbers of children being labeled as delayed when uncorrected ages were used. The authors concluded by stating that two age lines should be computed using the DDST. These age lines should represent both the corrected and the uncorrected age. Thus the examiner will have access to both sources of information when making judgments on developmental adequacy following DDST administration.

In my experience, correction for prematurity should be carried out until the child reaches 12 to 15 months of age. This is doubly important for those children who have experienced a particularly precarious neonatal period characterized by multiple complications and a lengthy stay in an intensive care nursery. One alternative available to the assessor is to chart developmental performance and change using both corrected and uncorrected ages. The assessor then has the information necessary to make decisions regarding developmental adequacy with both of these views in mind. Determining whether the need to correct for prematurity in these cases is due to prematurity alone, or to the additive effects of illness and hospitalization, may not be possible because of inherent difficulty in controlling multiple variables. However, given the precarious nature of prediction based on tests administered in infancy and on the serious nature of lost environmental opportunity for sick premature children, correcting for prematurity until 12 to 15 months of age is of value to the infant-toddler assessor (Palisano, Short, and Nelson, 1985).

SIGNIFICANCE OF CATCH-UP GROWTH

Only through serial assessment (reevaluation on a regular basis) does it become apparent that the significance of catch-up growth increases as the need to correct for prematurity lessens. Catch-up growth occurs when a child is less than 12 to 15 months of age, and the need to correct for prematurity decreases due to the child's display of more age-appropriate behavior. Catch-up growth may be defined as an accelerated rate of developmental skill mastery, thus reducing the gap between where the child is functioning and where he or she should be functioning. The degree of developmental delay that is detected following initial assessment is of particular importance when subsequent evaluations are completed. Initial test results serve as the basis for comparisons of future results. For the astute assessor, monitoring the presence of catch-up growth a child displays can be used to form opinions on developmental expectations.

The following example delineates the importance of monitoring catch-up growth through serial assessment. Consider a 6-month-old child with a history of prematurity (eight weeks) requiring a stay in an intensive care nursery of approximately eight weeks. If correction for prematurity takes place, as it should for a child younger than the 12 to 15 months previously specified, the child's 6 months' chronologic age would be considered as 4 months for developmental comparison purposes. If the child scores at the four-month level, then interpretation of assessment results would indicate that developmental progress is essentially normal. Thus a two-month developmental gap exists when comparing overall performance to chronologic age expectations. However, the noted gap is not viewed in an overly critical manner because of the process of correcting for prematurity.

As the child is assessed at later dates, however, and as the need to correct for prematurity is decreased, the degree of developmental gap should decrease. Hence catch-up growth is said to take place. If at 12 months of age the child scores at the 11-month level (recall that gestational age was 32 weeks), it can be said that catch-up growth has taken place because the child is approximately four weeks closer to displaying age-appropriate behavior regardless of correcting for prematurity. If the child displays age-appropriate behavior at subsequent evaluations (e.g., at 16 months) it is obvious that catch-up growth is complete and that an apparently normal sequence of developmental skill mastery is in place.

The rate and significance of catch-up growth has received little systematic study. Hanks (1987) attempted to measure catch-up growth in a cohort of 12 infants with a history of prematurity. The rate of catch-up growth was measured for the children through 18 months of age. These rates were compared with performance on later cognitive measures at 4 to 6 years of age. Although no significant correlation between the rate of catch-up growth and later performance was detected, child-by-child analysis of the data revealed that those children who earlier displayed a faster catch-up growth rate did somewhat better at 4 to 6 years of age. Perhaps correlations between catch-up growth and developmental performance at younger ages (3 to 4 years) may have revealed a stronger relationship between catch-up growth and later developmental performance in the Hanks study.

It may be that catch-up growth is more or less significant for various sub-populations within the premature population. As has been pointed out by a variety of investigators, the premature population is not a homogeneous group, since great variety exists concerning medical history secondary to prematurity (Rossetti, 1986; DeHirsh, Jansky, and Langford, 1966; Davies, 1981; Vohr and Oh, 1983). This variety, which was certainly present in the Hanks study, may have been the chief reason a more definite correlation between measures of catch-up growth and later developmental performance was not detected.

It seems reasonable to assume that an infant who maintains a developmental delay over time, or for whom the gap between present performance and age-appropriate performance widens, would carry a less favorable prognosis. On the other hand, if an infant displays a developmental delay based on uncorrected age on early test administrations but subsequently displays rapid catch-up growth with no delay noted at 12 to 15 months of age (no need to correct for prematurity), a more favorable prognosis is possible. Both corrected and uncorrected age scores are necessary to monitor catch-up growth. The experienced assessor uses measures of catch-up growth for both the premature and full-term infant to judge developmental adequacy and expectations. As previously noted, prediction based on early test administration is tenuous at best. However, using indexes of catch-up growth should assist the examiner in better understanding change over time and the significance of that change for long-term developmental achievement.

NEED FOR SERIAL ASSESSMENT

The previous discussion regarding catch-up growth pointed out that regular reevaluations are needed for making appropriate statements concerning developmental performance. Inherent in that discussion is the need for serial reevaluations of infants' and toddlers' developmental performance levels. A variety of questions regarding reevaluations arise, such as when assessment should begin, how frequently it should take place, what are the overall advantages of serial assessment, and how should the results of a single test administration be viewed?

Perhaps Kagan (1971) has suggested the best possible way in which results of infant assessment should be viewed. He indicated that each of the infants' and toddlers' responses — smiling, vocalizing, looking time, heart rate increases and decreases, and any other behaviors called for in infant assessment tests — are analogous to windows on a house. Each window gives the viewer a different glimpse into the contents of the house. To provide a coherent and complete picture of the interior of the home, it is necessary to gain as many points of view as possible. In many ways, past descriptions of infant-toddler assessment have not recognized the need to glimpse samples of child behavior repeatedly. Several important suggestions are provided by McCarthy (1980) on the need for regular and systematic infant-toddler assessment. These are listed in modified form:

1. In a testing situation the examiner is only able to elicit a limited sample of the child's behavior at best. If the examiner cannot feel reasonably confident about the sample elicited, it should not be quantified or labeled but simply described.
2. The younger the child, the less reliable predictions will be across the developmental dimensions mentioned.
3. Time, spontaneous recovery of function, and maturation are on the side of the young child and may make liars out of the best assessment tools.

These suggestions imply that the only way for the examiner to feel somewhat confident about the samples of behavior elicited is to gain reliable samples over time. Hence, serial assessment is mandatory. Murphy, Nichter, and Liden (1982) summarize the benefits of serial assessment in the following manner:

1. Serial assessment provides the only means of measuring developmental patterns and rates of development and change.
2. Serial assessment assists the practitioner in making decisions about intervention.
3. Serial assessment assists the practitioner in making decisions about the progress of interventions.
4. Serial assessment is the only means of detecting and monitoring new problems as the child matures.

These points imply that changes in development occur with time. Thus, it is imperative to monitor the child's development with serial observations. Determining if the child is steadily progressing in all areas of functioning, or if some areas are beginning to show delay or dysfunction, can only be accomplished through repeated observations. For infants and toddlers who are at mild risk, good serial observations entail routine developmental evaluations. For children with known developmental pathology, or those at higher risk of displaying developmental pathology, a more comprehensive schedule of evaluations may be indicated.

WHEN TO INITIATE ASSESSMENT ACTIVITY

At what age to begin initial assessment is the first question the assessor must face. No clear-cut formula fits each infant or toddler. Consequently, the assessor must address a variety of factors in making this decision: (1) concerns about the purpose of the assessment, (2) the setting in which the assessment activity will take place, (3) the referral source, (4) parental resources and willingness to participate in early assessment, (5) individual characteristics of the child, (6) medical history, (7) which test instruments to use, and (8) the need for support personnel.

For the practitioner working in a medical setting (particularly if the setting includes an intensive care nursery), initial assessment activity may take place before the child's discharge from the hospital. Data gained at an early age prove helpful as baseline information when subsequent evaluations are conducted. However, the assessor must be aware of the limitations inherent in assessment at such early ages. These limitations relate to the infant's overall state (see the next section), the nature of the setting itself, and the instruments used for infant assessment. The child has limited opportunity to interact with the environment in a normal manner during hospitalization, and thus behavioral responses obtained at an early age, especially for those children with an involved medical history, must be viewed with caution. At the very least, the practitioner employed in a medical setting should observe the child before discharge. Whether those observations include the administration of specific assessment instruments is up to the practitioner. The assessor may choose to make initial notes regarding environmental interaction and behavioral responses for a particular infant and use these observations when later, more formal assessment is undertaken.

For the practitioner working outside of a hospital setting, initial assessment will likely take place at a later date. This depends in part on the source of referral. The initial referral may be delayed until a deficit is suspected by parents or others involved in care of the child. This age may be delayed to an even greater degree if the child has not experienced a difficult medical course at or following birth. However, for children with known risk for developmental pathology due to medical factors, assessment outside the medical setting may not be delayed to the same degree.

The impact on parents of having a premature or medically fragile child cannot be underestimated. Thus, parents may need some time to make early adaptations and develop adequate parenting skills before the initiation of assessment activity. Parental willingness to participate in infant-toddler assessment may be an additional factor to consider when evaluating the age at which initial assessment activity should take place. Practitioners should be in frequent contact with parents in an attempt to gauge the best time to initiate appropriate evaluative measures. Parents usually are most receptive to followup efforts if they are informed of the value of these efforts from a preventive standpoint. Parental concerns such as time involvement, cost, and other issues are more easily dealt with if parents understand the need and value of assessment and follow-up. If the parents understand that the assessor is interested in ensuring optimal development for their child and that early and regular assessment is an integral part of the process, they will more than likely be quite supportive of regular evaluation appointments.

Individual child characteristics will also play an important role in determining when to initiate assessment. For the child who has been through a particularly difficult neonatal period, the need to initiate appropriate activity is much stronger and should take place soon after the parental adjustment issues are near completion. If the examiner is aware that a child is being discharged to a home setting that is less than optimal, even in the absence of severe neonatal complications, early assessment may be desirable. The assessor should be apprised of the neonatal history, as well as potential sequelae based on known risk factors to make accurate decisions on initiating assessment activity.

An additional factor that must be considered in determining when to initiate assessment activity relates to the need for support personnel as well as the content of assessment appointments. If the practitioner wishes to perform a complete evaluative workup of a child, and if the evaluation is part of a comprehensive neonatal follow-up program that involves a variety of other professionals, then the start of formal assessment procedures may be delayed until the child has been in the home setting for 1 to 3 months. One must also consider that the more people involved with the infant or toddler, the greater the potential for delay because of logistical considerations regarding schedules and time.

In regard to the factors specified above, it becomes difficult to identify a specific age at which early assessment activity should commence. The actual age of the child may vary in light of a host of considerations. The overriding concern is that the assessment process begin at the earliest possible age. In my experience, the initiation of assessment activity should begin, if at all possible, within the first 3 months after birth. Data gained during this initial evaluation, even in light of the variables that render observations in these early months tenuous for many children, can constitute important baseline information to which later assessment results may be compared. Baseline assessment data are imperative if measures of catch-up growth and child change are to be used in making various decisions regarding programming and future needs of infants and toddlers.

ASSESSMENT INTERVALS

Following initial assessment and all subsequent evaluations, the assessor must determine the best schedule for future assessment activity. The question of how often a particular child should be seen for developmental follow-up is not an easy one to answer. No set formula for frequency of assessment exists. However, a number of variables are important to consider. These variables relate in large measure to medical history, age, infant-toddler performance, whether the child is receiving early intervention services, the number of other professionals involved in follow-up and intervention, variables in the child's home setting, and unanticipated factors relating to health.

Perhaps the initial factors to keep in mind when determining intervals between visits relate to a combination of the child's age and performance on administered developmental instruments. Keep in mind that the younger the child, the greater the potential for change from evaluation to evaluation. For example, if a child is evaluated before hospital discharge and, based on behavioral observations, is felt to be at moderate to high risk for developmental pathology, the frequency of visits for follow-up activity might be every three months. Thus, the child might be evaluated as many as four times within the first year. If at initial assessment the child is observed to display behavior that is close to age expectations, contact with the parents may be maintained but formal reevaluation delayed until six months later. However, as a general rule of thumb, if the practitioner detects behavior that suggests a developmental pathology, an assessment schedule of follow-up every three months is recommended (Rossetti, 1986). The three-month schedule allows parents and other professionals time to implement early intervention activities as well as time for the child to benefit from such activity.

The infant's medical history may also dictate the frequency of follow-up visits. For those children who have experienced serious neonatal complications with known relationships to later neurologic and cognitive sequelae, more frequent evaluations might be indicated. Likewise, infants at increased risk due to environmental factors might be seen more frequently. If the assessor realizes that a particular child may be lost to follow-up, all efforts should be made to determine as best as possible the child's developmental performance, and appropriate attempts to initiate intervention should be undertaken. A schedule of reassessment every three months for the first year of life would appear to be appropriate in these instances. Based on the child's status during the first year, this schedule can be readily altered if necessary.

After the child's first year the schedule of visits may be altered. If optimum observational opportunities have been afforded the assessor throughout the first year, then a fairly comprehensive picture of the child's developmental progress over time has been obtained. Data of this nature are indispensable in formulating future suggestions. Recall that one question the assessor should always attempt to answer is, "What next?" One outcome of posing that question relates to when the child should next be seen as developmental change is gauged and monitored. If accurate descriptions of developmental status are to be made, systematic and detailed observations of child performance starting at an early age are essential. In the absence of systematic assessment of this nature, developmental pathology cannot be detected, early intervention cannot be initiated, and optimal skill acquisition may not be achieved.

DETERMINATION OF INFANT STATE

The practitioner who has any degree of experience in assessing and measuring developmental competence for infants and toddlers is acutely aware that infant-toddler performance on a given test is significantly affected by the particular state (level of consciousness or arousal) the child displays during test administration. One question the examiner should pose following the administration of any assessment instrument — formal or informal — relates to whether the sample of behavior obtained truly represented the child's potential or if it was altered by other factors. This, in essence, is a reliability question, and the astute examiner interprets observed behavior in light of the implications of this question. Following each assessment it might be wise to ask the caregiver whether the behaviors displayed by the child during the assessment reflected the child's true abilities. In other words, does the child display behaviors at home or in other settings that were not present during the evaluation? If so, what were they, and how long have these behaviors been noted by the caregiver? Certainly one factor that must be considered when evaluating the reliability of observed behaviors has to do with infant state.

Infant state can be defined as the level of alertness and environmental interaction patterns present in an infant or toddler at a given point. Brazelton (1973) was one of the first investigators to discuss the importance of considering infant states when observing normal, healthy newborns. The child's reactions to stimuli during test administration must therefore be interpreted within the context of the particular state of consciousness the child is in at a given point. As a result, the child's responses may vary according to state. State depends on physiologic variables such as hunger, nutrition, degree of hydration, and the time within the wake-sleep cycle the assessment is conducted. The concept of state has been applied most readily to infants (under 6 months of age). However, the concept of environmental interaction and factors that influence responsiveness to test stimuli is equally important for children in the 1-to-3 year age range even though there is less written regarding state measurement for children in this age range. For the assessor working with children from birth to 6 months of age, particularly if the child has an involved medical history involving prematurity, low birth weight, and associated complications, an understanding of state is important for more accurate interpretation of assessment results.

An additional concept regarding state is that state status is quite flexible and changes readily. As Brazelton (1973) has indicated, the pattern of states as well as the movement from one state to another appear to be important characteristics of infants in the neonatal period, and this kind of evaluation may be the best predictor of the infant's receptivity and ability to respond to stimuli in a cognitive sense. Table 4-1 summarizes infant state descriptions provided by Brazelton relative to healthy newborns (Brazelton, 1973). As is readily evident, the examiner would not expect to obtain good samples of environmental interaction during several states in which environmental interest is less than optimal.

The application of the concept of infant state to premature infants is a more recent development and would certainly impact assessment activity performed on children in this category. Gorski, Davison, and Brazelton (1979) presented an insightful description of the stages of behavioral organization that the assessor might expect to observe while the child is yet in the hospital. Basically three stages of behavioral organization were described by Gorski's group. It is imperative that the assessor be aware of these as assessment activity is undertaken with children younger than 6 months of age who present an involved medical history due to prematurity and associated complications or other medically significant factors. Unlike the states described above, the states listed below are better viewed as stages. This is because the stressed infant is unlikely to show as much flex-

TABLE 4-1. Infant states

State	*Characteristics*
Sleep state	
Deep sleep	Deep sleep with regular breathing, no activity, no eye movement
Light sleep	Rapid eye movements, random startle movements, sucking movements off and on
Awake state	
Drowsy, semidozing	Eyes opened or closed, eyelids fluttering, movements usually smooth, mild startling noted
Alert	Bright looks, focuses attention on objects, motor activity at minimum
Eyes open	Considerable motor activity, increase in startling, high activity level
Crying	Intense crying, difficult to break through even with novel stimulation

Source: Adapted from T. Brazelton (1973). Neonatal behavior assessment scale. Philadelphia: J.B. Lippincott.

ibility in short periods as is the healthy newborn. During the final two stages described below, it is more likely that the assessor will observe behaviors more reflective of the states presented in Table 4-1. The length of time an infant will remain in any of the stages presented below depends on a number of factors; however, the overriding concern is the infant's overall medical status. The stages described by Gorski's group are as follows:

1. *In-turning or physiologic stage.* During the usual course of events for the stressed premature infant, normal environmental interaction with caregivers that leads to the establishment of a bond resulting in mutually satisfying interaction is not possible. The premature infant must first develop sufficient physical integrity and internal stability before being able to use caregiver support and input needed to make continuous developmental gains. Simply stated, the ill infant is not able to benefit fully from interaction with caregivers durng the early period following birth because the infant's energy is directed toward surviving and maintaining physiologic stability. The assessor who is employed in a hospital setting with access to the intensive care nursery must be aware of the limitations inherent in attempting to observe behavior while the child is in the in-turned state. The infant during this state is quite sick and cannot pay attention, much less respond in an appropriate manner, to the type of stimuli to which he or she is likely to be exposed during a standard developmental assessment. Even the process of observing performance must be undertaken with the implicit understanding that the bulk of the infant's energy is directed inward.

2. *Coming out.* The child now has mastered a minimum capacity to control and maintain physiologic systems. He or she must now begin to build on these basic organizational patterns. This stage represents the first active response to the environment and implies a more active response to outside stimuli, both nutritional and social. This is the period when changes in the caregiver environment have an important impact on the child's physical well being and growth. It is at this time that initial attachment to a primary caregiver is established and strengthened. This is the period when the mother's presence can be helpful to both baby and mother as the baby is showing some awareness of the world and those in it. This second stage of environmental awareness is usually experienced by the child while he or she is still a patient in the intensive care nursery. This period spans the time from when the child is no longer acutely ill and is able to breathe effectively and to absorb enough calories to gain weight to when the baby can be dismissed from the hospital. This is a time when behavioral observations can point to caregiver interactions that can foster the infant's physical as well as social-interactive development. Any observations of behavioral competence during this period must be made with the knowledge that this is the first time the infant is displaying a greater awareness of the environment and is initially attempting to interact with it.

3. *Reciprocity.* This is the ultimate state of environmental opportunity. At this point the infant is strong enough to breathe, feed, and respond to caregiver behaviors in specific and predictable ways. This stage may begin sometime before hospital discharge and continue after the infant is in the home setting. It is also possible that in some instances this stage may not fully begin until after the child has been in the home setting for several weeks or longer. Once this stage begins, the infant still faces the task of overcoming any remaining problems associated with the intial illness. The emerging relationships between caregiver and infant play a central role during this stage. It is important to recall that the infant's ability or inability to interact with the environment in a reciprocal manner may be an important precursor to developmental skill acquisition at later stages of skill maturation. The infant who is unable to demonstrate initial interest in the environment may be displaying behaviors that indicate increased potential for developmental pathology.

It quickly becomes obvious to the assessor that regardless of the age at which the infant or toddler is assessed, particular attention must be paid to the child's state. For the examiner to disregard state when interpreting assessment results is to set oneself up for inaccurate impressions and judgments about developmental skill mastery.

One assessment instrument that pays particular attention to the manner in which the infant or toddler responds during test administration is the *Bayley Scales of Infant Development* (Bayley, 1969). Following administration of the mental and motor portions of the Bayley, the infant behavior record is administered. A variety of areas are assessed, with the examiner judging how the child responded on the mental and motor scales. The infant behavior scale requires the examiner to rate 16 areas relative to infant-toddler response patterns. Table 4-2 lists the areas subjectively evaluated by the examiner in an attempt to gauge the reliability of the responses provided by the child.

Favorable and positive responses in each of these areas assist the examiner in determining if the samples of behavior elicited more or less indicated the child's true abilities. Although the infant behavior record accompanies the Bayley scale, the patterns of performance that it directs attention toward should prove helpful regardless of the specific assessment instrument employed by the examiner.

In essence, regardless of the child's age, the examiner must be alert to factors that influence the reliability of the samples of infant-toddler behavior elicited. Recalling that the samples obtained represent how the child did only on the day of test administration should signficantly reinforce the need for serial evaluation as previously outlined. The state the child is in at any given point is influenced by factors within the child's environment as well as within the child's constitution. These factors can interact in powerful

TABLE 4-2. Infant behavior scale: Areas assessed

1. Social orientation: Responsiveness to people, mother, examiner
2. Cooperativeness: Cooperates with examiner
3. Fearfulness: Reaction to new situations
4. Tension: Tenseness of body
5. General emotional tone: Degree of happiness
6. Object orientation: Responsiveness to objects, imaginative play with objects, attachment to objects
7. Goal directedness: Persistence in goal-directed efforts
8. Attention span: Persistence in attending to any one object, activity, person
9. Endurance: Behavior constancy
10. Activity: Amount of gross body movements
11. Reactivity: Sensitivity or excitability
12. Sensory areas of interest: Sights, sounds, noisemaking, manipulating, mouthing
13. Energy and coordination: Level of energy and coordination for age
14. Judgment of test: Optimal versus minimal adequacy of test results as indicator of child's ability
15. Unusual or deviant behavior: Any unusual or deviant behavior
16. General evaluation: Normal or exceptional child performance

Source: Adapted from N. Bayley (1969). Bayley scales of infant development. New York: Psychological Corporation.

ways, potentially altering the child's ability to demonstrate patterns of environmental interaction that accurately reflect developmental skill acquisition.

ASSESSING ATYPICAL INFANTS AND TODDLERS

The developmental assessment of infants and toddlers with a moderate to severe degree of developmental pathology presents the examiner with a unique set of circumstances. On one hand, the presence of developmental delay is not in question because the child may have a history reflecting medical-environmental factors related to the delay noted. On the other hand, the examiner's goal is to obtain accurate indexes of cognitive ability in the presence of limited ability on the infant's part to display reliable samples of behavior consistently. The examiner may experience frustration in such instances. The frustration arises from several sources but most prominently from the inability of assessment tools to meet the needs of this population readily.

Many assessors have completed developmental evaluations of such children only to feel that the child had better overall developmental ability than was revealed by formal assessment results. Zelazo (1982) has noted that many assessors sense, through clinical judgment sharpened by years of experience, that a particular child has greater awareness of the environment than formal tests may reveal. The examiner may have detected several subtle behaviors that lead to this conclusion. Thus, the assessor is left with a haunting feeling that there is something wrong with traditional methods of developmental assessment, particularly for this population of children. The feeling that there must be a better way of assessing developmental ability among children with serious developmental delay is a major source of frustration for the assessor.

Because children with developmental pathology are evaluated on tests that were standardized on normal populations of children, the results often yield a depressed estimate of the child's general develomental skill acquisition. This is as it should be, however, since the purpose of the instrument is to detect delayed patterns of development when compared with children displaying age-appropriate developmental skill mastery. However, little is known about what constitutes a normal pattern of abnormal development, or even if such a pattern exists.

Behaviors measured on infant tests may have little direct correspondence to intellectual development. Although test construction has been undertaken with the notion that the behaviors elicited correlate with cognitive ability at one point, little empirical data exist to support such a supposition. In other words, how readily do some of the tasks expected on infant-toddler tests correlate with actual levels of cognitive ability? If the actual correlation is not strong (current instruments have assumed that it is strong), then what can be assumed about the child who is unable to demonstrate certain behaviors due to motor deficits or other sensory impairments? Is it possible that false assumptions regarding such a child's developmental skill mastery will be made? The use of conventional testing procedures with developmentally disabled children almost invariably places their developmental status in doubt. This is much more so for the child with enhanced developmental delay.

On the basis of the previous discussion, it is imperative that the examiner develop an overall philosophy and methodology to employ when assessing atypical children. Methodology in assessing atypical children will vary between examiners depending on level of experience and comfort in altering set and standard assessment techinques. In other words, the examininer may need to be alert to patterns of behavior that reveal nonstandard samples of developmental ability and yet that do not constitute behaviors easily noted on normed assessment instruments. The precise patterns of behavior that the examiner should be alert to include the following.

Developmental Auditory Behavior

Response patterns to auditory stimuli are related to chronologic age and general patterns of development. A sufficient database exists on normal patterns of interaction with auditory stimuli for healthy and normally developing infants and toddlers. An insufficient database exists regarding how infants and toddlers who have a developmental delay react to various auditory stimuli. Certainly, children with known hearing impairment would be expected to display aberrant patterns of response. However, children without impaired hearing who are developmentally delayed likewise may display patterns of response that differentiate them from children with appropriate developmental performance. Several patterns of aberrant response to auditory stimuli might include the following:*

1. *Excessive tuning out.* Some children may display behaviors that reflect excessive tuning out of sound. These patterns may be in excess of those that would reflect normal adaptation to sound.
2. *Delayed response.* Response latency may be greater in developmentally delayed children; that is, developmentally delayed children may display awareness of auditory stimuli in a manner that shows late awareness of sound.
3. *Strength of response.* The strength of response to auditory stimuli that are above the child's threshold may not be different from response strength to auditory stimuli closer to the child's hearing threshold for children displaying developmental pathology.

Rossetti and Kyle (1988) presented data supporting the relationship between aberrant patterns of response to auditory stimuli and performance on global development assessment instruments. In the Rossetti and Kile study, correlations were obtained between indexes of auditory behavior and scores on the Bayley Scales of Infant Development. Results revealed that children who scored below age expectations on the Bayley scales also displayed deviant responses to auditory stimuli as judged by a team of audiologists observing the child's response to the auditory stimuli presented. The monitoring of auditory behavior and its relationship to developmental pathology is an area that has received little systematic investigation. At the very least, it behooves the assessor to pay special attention to patterns of response a child may exhibit when exposed to familiar and unfamiliar auditory stimuli.

Problem Solving

Some existing assessment tools pay attention to the child's problem-solving ability during test administration. One example of a problem-

* J. Kile, personal communication, March 21, 1989.

solving opportunity afforded a child during the administration of the Bayley Scales of Infant Development involves the child's being given a doll that is missing its head. The child is given both parts (body and head). The examiner is instructed to observe whether the child spontaneously places the head on top of the body. Other examples of problem-solving opportunities relate to form board completion and test items that require a child to find an object that is placed out of visual contact (e.g., under a piece of cloth). It is more likely, however, that spontaneous problem solving may take place that is not part of the formal assessment. The examiner must be alert to these spontaneously occurring events. The exact form this activity may take is quite varied. It may be that the child demonstrates task learning or that objects are used in a novel manner. Examples of this type of behavior might include the child's determining how to open a latched box in an attempt to secure toys or opening the mother's diaper bag to secure a bottle or other object. Whatever form problem solving may assume, it is important for the assessor to note and describe the event.

Environmental Awareness

Once assessment activity is initiated, it quickly becomes obvious whether the child is displaying sufficient levels of environmental awareness. Environmental awareness is in part related to the state the child is in at a given point. For example, during the in-turned state (while the child is in the intensive care nursery), little if any environmental awareness is evidenced. In fact, in most instances the child is sensory satiated and will not register awareness of even noxious stimuli. During a crying, agitated, or drowsy-sleep state, it is unlikely that the child will display appropriate awareness of environmental stimuli.

Once the examiner believes that the child's awareness of the environment should result in certain behaviors or response patterns, noting environmental awareness becomes important. A lack of awareness regarding new situations, people, events, and interactions is instructive to the examiner as a barometer of the degree of general alertness the child displays. For children with moderate to severe developmental delay, degree of alertness is important, since it may be one of the primary means the examiner has to determine develomental adequacy in light of sensory handicaps. Environmental awareness relates as well to the child's response to new or novel stimuli. If no variations are seen in the presence of new stimuli, questions arise about the child's overall level of alertness.

Desire for New Stimuli and Experiences

Some children, even those with serious motor or sensory deficits, display behaviors that indicate a hunger for environmental interaction and experience. The child who demonstrates little or no interest in the world around, even during times of quiet and relative overall physiologic stability, is telling the examiner a great deal about cognitive processes in operation at that point. The desire for new stimuli and experiences will certainly be altered by the child's state.

A child's desire for environmental experience may take a variety of forms. These may include active visual exploration of the surroundings, acute awareness of auditory stimuli, interest in exploring novel tactile objects, and an overall indication that the child is hungry to learn and be exposed to new things. These behaviors may be observed even in instances where sensory handicaps exist. Take, for example, the child at 28 months of age who is not yet walking. It is possible that even in light of the lack of independent locomotion, the child will make attempts to secure objects either independently or with assistance from caregivers. In instances where the child shows little or no desire to interact with the environment, questions must be raised about the degree to which this lack of environmental hunger suggests a potential cognitive deficit.

Manipulative Behavior

One indicator the examiner should be aware of relates to attempts the child makes to manipulate or control the test environment. This may include attempts to manipulate people or the situation in general. The actual forms this behavior may take include crying, whining, avoiding exposure to new stimuli, and avoiding eye contact. Fearful responses to new situations and people are not unusual. However, if this pattern persists and is present even after sufficient opportunity has been given the child to gain familiarity with the test setting and the examiner, some form of manipulative behavior should be suspected. In the presence of these behaviors the examiner should not automatically assume the child is not able to perform the desired activity. Rather, the examiner should try to determine to what degree, if any, the behaviors reflect the child's attempt to control the situation. These patterns are usually not seen in children under 15 to 18 months of age. In essence, behaviors of this nature reflect the child's desire to control on his or her terms. Persistent behaviors of this nature reflect the fact that the child is making an attempt to control the assessment situation consciously.

Meaningful Interaction with the Environment

Children display various patterns of interaction with the environment. Some of these patterns are appropriate, while others reflect less than optimal interaction strategies. The child who manipulates objects in a random manner is displaying nonmeaningful behavior that should be described by the assessor. For example, when given a toy car or truck, the 18-month-old child is likely to push it along the floor in an appropriate manner. The child may even include noises, thus indicating an understanding of meaningful play with the toy. When given a cup and spoon, the 12-month-old child may choose to perform stirring or eating actions with the spoon. On the other hand, if the child is presented with a crayon and a piece of paper, behaviors such as mouthing (appropriate at ages under 9 months), throwing the object, or a general lack of understanding regarding the function of the crayon may be noted. These patterns may be present at all times or on a variable basis. Behavior of this nature is important because it is an indicator of the child's deficiencies in cognitive integration and previous sensory experience. It may reflect inadequate exposure to the environment or a depressed ability to benefit from environmental opportunity. Certainly at ages above 18 months interactional patterns with the environment can serve as an important barometer of the child's overall developmental ability and potential.

*   *   *

What the preceding list of behaviors points to is that during any examination, particularly an examination with an infant or toddler with moderate to severe developmental delay, the assessor must pay special attention to indexes of developmental level that are not traditionally part of standardized assessment instruments. Although the examiner's ability to quantify these behaviors is limited, their presence can be noted and described in detail. One general principle to keep in mind during the assessment process is that events will take place that are outside of the standard and routine. Infants and toddlers may not respond to test stimuli in desired ways. It is crucial that the examiner not miss the significance of the patterns of behavior noted above. Hence, the examiner must be prepared to delineate these events without quantifying or interpreting them. Simple description of the behaviors is all that is needed at times. Over time, as subsequent evaluations are conducted, the examiner will have a rich source of observations to assist in determining developmental progress and change. The skills necessary to make observations of this nature come with experience and the willingness to learn from the infants and toddlers who are the recipients of assessment activity. Conventional tests pose substantial problems for children with developmental disabilities. The examiner must be alert to these problems and have strategies in mind to compensate for them.

SUMMARY

A variety of issues concerning infant-toddler assessment have been raised in this chapter. The discussion is intended to sharpen the examiner's understanding of obvious as well as not-so-obvious considerations of infant-toddler assessment. The process is by no means a clear-cut one. Rather, it involves a philosophy of assessment that places the examiner in the position of learner. As such, it is imperative that the assessor develop acute observational skills that assist in eliciting behaviors on which to judge the child's developmental skill level. A host of decisions rest on data of these nature. The children served deserve optimal opportunities to demonstrate maximal skill learning during the preschool years. Accurate assessment is in large measure the starting point of this process.

STUDY QUESTIONS

1. A variety of issues were raised in this chapter regarding why infants and toddlers should be the recipients of assessment activity. Discuss these issues.
2. Define assessment.
3. How predictive are tests administered in early childhood for later performance? What factors must the assessor keep in mind regarding the interpretation of assessment results?
4. What is meant by the term *infant state?* How might infant state behavior alter assessment results?
5. Assessing atypical infants and toddlers is one of the biggest challenges the practitioner will face. What behaviors might the assessor use in assisting in the assessment process?

REFERENCES

Brazelton, T. (1973). *Neonatal behavior assessment scale.* Philadelphia: J.B. Lippincott.
Bayley, N. (1969). *Bayley scales of infant development.* New York: Psychological Corporation.
Coplan, J. (1982). Parental estimate of child's developmental level in a high risk population. *American Journal of Disorders in Childhood, 136,* 101.
Davies, D. (1981). Growth for small for date babies. *Early Human Development, 5,* 95.
DeHirsh, K., Jansky, J., & Langford, W. (1966). Comparisons between prematurely and maturely born children at three age levels. *American Journal of Orthopsychiatry, 36,* 616.
Elliman, A., Bryan, E., Elliman, A. D., & Dubowitz, L. (1985). Denver developmen-

tal screening test and preterm infants. *Archives of Disease in Children, 60,* 20.

Escalona, S. (1982). Babies at double hazard: Early development of infants at biologic and social risk. *Pediatrics, 70,* 670.

Gorski, P., Davidson, M., & Brazelton, T. (1979). Stages of behavioral organization in the high-risk neonate: Theoretical and clinical considerations. *Seminars in Perinatology, 3,* 61.

Hack, M., Merkatz, I., McGrath, S., Jones, P., & Fanaroff, A. (1984). Catch-up growth in very-low-birth-weight infants. *American Journal of Disease in Children, 138,* 370.

Hanks, J. (1987). The ability of catch-up growth to predict later cognitive and language performance in high risk infants. Unpublished master's thesis. Northeast Missouri State University, Kirksville, MO.

Hunt, J. (1981). Predicting intelligence disorders in childhood for preterm infants born with birth weights below 1501 grams. In S. Friedman and M. Sigman (Eds.), *Preterm birth and psychological development.* New York: Academic Press.

Hunt, J., & Rhodes, L. (1977). Mental development of preterm infants during the first year. *Child Development. 48,* 204.

Kagan, L. (1971). *Change and continuity in infancy.* New York: John Wiley & Sons.

McCarthy, J. (1980). Assessment of young children with learning problems: Beyond the paralysis of analysis. In E. Sell (Ed.), *Follow-up of the high-risk newborn: A practical approach.* Springfield, MA: Charles C Thomas.

McCall, R., Hogarty, P., & Hurlbut, N. (1972). Transitions in infancy sensory motor development and the prediction of childhood I.Q. *American Psychologist, 27,* 728.

McCormick, M., Shapiro, S., & Starfield, B. (1982). Factors associated with maternal opinion of infant development. Clues to the vulnerable child, *Pediatrics, 69,* 537.

Miller, G., Dubowitz, L., & Palmer, P. (1984). Follow-up of preterm infants: Is correction of the developmetal quotient for prematurity helpful? *Early Human Development, 9,* 137.

Murphy, T., Nichter, C., & Liden, C. (1982). Developmental outcome of the high-risk infant: A review of methodological issues. *Seminars in Perinatology, 6,* 4.

Palisano, R., Short, M., & Nelson, D. (1985). Chronological age vs. adjusted age in assessing motor development of healthy twelve-month-old premature and full-term infants. *Physical and Occupational Therapy in Pediatrics, 5,* 1.

Parents of infants and young children. (1986). University of Illinois, Department of Speech and Hearing Science.

Rossetti, L. (1986). *High risk infants: Identification, assessment, and intervention.* Austin, TX: PRO-ED.

Rossetti, L., & Kile, J. (1988). Neurodevelopmental assessment of infants and toddlers. Paper presented at the annual convention of the American Speech-Language-Hearing Association, Boston, MA.

Siegel, L. (1983). Correction for prematurity and its consequences for the assessment of the very low birth weight infant. *Child Development, 54,* 1174.

Siegel, L. (1981). Infant tests as predictors of cognitive and language development at two years. *Child Development, 52,* 545.

Siegel, L. (1979). Infant perceptual, cognitive, and motor behaviors as predictors of subsequent cognitive and language development. *Canadian Journal of Psychology, 33,* 382.

Vohr, B. & Oh, W. (1983). Growth and development in preterm infants small for gestational age. *Journal of Pediatrics, 103,* 941.

Zelazo, P. (1982). Alternative assessment procedures for handicapped infants and toddlers. In D. Bricker (Ed.), *Intervention with at-risk and handicapped infants.* Baltimore: University Park Press.

Zelazo, P., Zelazo, R., & Kolb, S. (1972). Walking in the newborn, *Science, 176,* 314.

CHAPTER 5

Collecting and Reporting Assessment Data

Obtaining Case History
Information
    Questionnaires
    Direct Interview

Developmental Screening

Types of Assessment
Instruments
    Global Assessment Instruments
    Domain-Specific Assessment
        Instruments
    Norm-Referenced Assessment
        Instruments
    Criterion-Referenced
        Assessment Instruments

Developmental Log

Interpretation of Results

Communication of Assessment
Results
    Communication with Parents
    Communication with Other
        Professionals

Summary

Study Questions

References

Once basic pretest considerations have been dealt with and the assessor is in a position to initiate assessment activity, different questions arise regarding various methods that may be used to collect assessment data. These issues relate to obtaining case history information, interviewing caregivers, types of assessment instruments, choosing appropriate assessment instruments, interpreting test results, and communicating results with appropriate persons. These are not easy issues to address, and in fact a variety of factors must be considered. These factors relate to the purpose of the assessment, the examiner's background and experience, the developmental domain to be assessed (specific developmental domain or overall developmental assessment), examiner familiarity with available assessment instruments, the setting of the assessment, whether the assessor is functioning alone or as a member of a team, the child's age, and the degree of potential developmental deficit present (determined from referral or case history information). There certainly is no shortage of assessment instruments from which to choose (see Appendix B). The question is, which test(s) should the assessor use? An additional issue to address is whether the activity that is directed toward the infant or toddler is designed to provide in-depth assessment information or is simply screening to detect potential developmental delay. These factors will, in large measure, direct which instruments to select and which other methods to employ.

OBTAINING CASE HISTORY INFORMATION

The preceding chapter introduced the pertinence of information, regardless of its source, about the infant or toddler. Certainly one of the richest sources of information, and one that should be explored before assessment activity is initiated, is accurate case history data. Such data are quite valuable because they provide a host of factors on which the examiner bases important decisions, including the actual selection of assessment instruments. Case history information may be obtained from two primary sources: questionnaires and direct interview of the caregivers.

QUESTIONNAIRES

Regardless of the employment setting, the professionals employed, the child's age, or any suspected developmental problem, it is common practice to gain information about the infant or toddler through the use of questionnaires. In most instances the questionnaire is sent to the caregivers before the assessment date. This allows the assessor to learn a little about the child before actually seeing the infant or toddler for formal assessment.

Using questionnaires to gather case history information has both advantages and disadvantages.

One of the disadvantages concerns the questions asked on the questionnaire. Of necessity, the question must be generic; that is, they must be stated in a manner that is likely to elicit responses regardless of a particular child's specific attributes. The questionnaire must be constructed with all possible respondents in mind. Hence, the actual questions tend to be somewhat ambiguous and may be more or less applicable for certain infants and toddlers.

A second disadvantage is that questions may engender guilt in the caregivers. If the caregiver exhibits any degree of reluctance in response accuracy, certain types of questions may elicit responses that are not wholly accurate. The assessor may then have inaccurate information, which may lead to inaccurate judgments about the child before assessment instruments are administered. In addition, parents may not always understand the questions posed, resulting in inaccurate information. The parents may have deficient reading skills, again resulting in inaccurate or incomplete information being supplied. A final disadvantage of the questionnaire is that questions, if answered in one particular manner, may prevent the respondent from providing any additional information. The result is that a less than accurate overall picture of the child is available to the assessor before the initiation of formal assessment activity.

Although these disadvantages exist, the use of some form of questionnaire is well established and certainly has a place as one tool available for gaining information about the infant or toddler. Appendix A presents a variety of questionnaires that the assessor may wish to use or adapt to fit specific needs. No matter how well constructed the questionnaire is, however, it should never take the place of a personal interview.

DIRECT INTERVIEW

A direct (intake) interview is one that is conducted before formal assessment activity is initiated. It is a conversation, directed by the assessor, that is carried out for specific purposes, such as gaining information about the child, determining caregiver attitudes concerning the child, and providing the assessor with an opportunity to determine the impact that the suspected developmental delay has had on the family unit. Figure 5-1 presents a sample format that the intake interview may follow. The intake interview differs from the interpretive interview that is conducted following assessment activity. The latter is designed to explain to the caregiver the results of the assessment and to answer any questions that may arise. A more complete discussion of the interpretive interview is presented later in this

AREAS TO BE COVERED	SAMPLE QUESTIONS

Biographical information	Date of birth
	Nature of problem
	    Who first suspected problem?
	    How long ago?
	    Times when it is better or worse?
	    Professionals already consulted?
	    What has been done already?
	    What do parents want from assessor?
	    Parent's view of problem

Medical history	Significant problems during pregnancy or delivery
	    Birth weight and gestational age
	    Prolonged hospitalization
	    Accidents, illness, or surgeries
	    Medications
	    Medical practitioners consulted
	    Results of previous medical evaluations

Developmental history	Developmental milestones across domains
	    Areas parents feel child is behind
	    Areas of strength and weakness
	    Developmental change over past several months

Educational history	Previous intervention provided
	    Results of previous intervention
	    Developmental domains worked on
	    Future educational programs

Social history	Number of siblings Opportunities with peers Interactional patterns with peers Behavioral or social problems Interactional patterns with adults Fearful behaviors Bizzare behaviors

Figure 5-1. Sample direct (intake) interview format.

chapter. Overall, there are at least three main goals the assessor should keep in mind when conducting intake interviews.

Goal One: Obtaining Information

Although it may seem obvious to the experienced assessor, it is worth restating that, as assessors, we must listen before we talk. Emerick (1969) has stated that there are three reasons why being a good listener aids the interview process. First, the assessor permits the caregiver an opportunity to talk out the suspected problem and to express fears and feelings. This enables the assessor to understand better the whole child in the context of the family. It also enables the assessor to realize more fully the sequence of events that have led to the point where the infant or toddler is before the actual assessment. A second benefit of listening is that the assessor is better able to gain an understanding of the type of information that the parents may need as part of the interpretive interview. A final benefit of careful listening during the intake interview is that the assessor is able to balance previous information obtained through the questionnaire (which may have resulted in the assessor's forming a preliminary opinion regarding the child) with the actual state of affairs.

Parents quickly learn the degree to which the assessor is really listening to what is being said. The wise assessor works at being a good listener and communicates to the parents in a variety of ways that what they have to say is important to the entire assessment process. It is important that the caregivers feel they are co-workers in the assessment process. This feeling is more easily accomplished if the assessor communicates interest and concern during the interview. In some instances the assessor may set a less-than-optimal tone early in the interactions with the parents. This can be difficult to overcome in later interactions.

The major portion of the intake interview is concerned with gaining information about the child's history. This is accomplished by the assessor's asking direct questions regarding important aspects of the infant or toddler. Perhaps the best way to initiate the interview is to ask the caregivers why they are seeking assessment services. The actual reasons may be obvious; however, it is instructive to hear the caregivers' response to that initial question. Although a variety of formats exist, the direct interview should cover at least five major areas concerning the child's past history. Questions should be directed toward (1) the history of the suspected developmental problem, (2) the child's developmental history, (3) the medical history, (4) the social-family history, and (5) the educational history.

The degree to which each of these areas is explored will depend on a variety of factors. These include the child's age, the presenting problem, the referring source, and the information obtained during the initial part of the interview. The experienced interviewer is able to determine which areas need in-depth exploration as the interview progresses. For example, if in response to questions concerning the child's medical history it becomes known that the child has a history of seizure activity, the interviewer will explore the medications and interventions taken to control the seizures. In essence, what transpires is a process in which the interviewer takes information during each stage of the interview and uses that information to determine the specific areas that require more detailed exploration. It is imperative that the interviewer be able to use information obtained during the interview to direct later interview questions. The ability to do so is enhanced through experience and practice as well as through observation of established interviewers.

Goal Two: Giving Information

Giving information relates to the examiner's being prepared to answer the caregivers' questions about the infant or toddler. In some instances, the caregivers may have had multiple opportunities to interact with other professionals in a position to answer relevant questions. In other instances, the caregivers may have had only minimal contact with other professionals before the assessment. The astute assessor should attempt to sense early in the interview how strongly the caregivers want their questions answered. Keep in mind that it is a mistake to provide too much information too early. That is to say, before the assessment activity is completed, the assessor should avoid making prognostic statements regarding either the child's present performance or future developmental potential. The assessor places himself or herself in a difficult position if these statements are made before assessment activity is completed.

Emerick (1969) describes six principles to keep in mind when imparting information to parents as part of an interview:

1. Be aware of the emotional static that may prevent the parents from really hearing the answers to the questions they pose.
2. Do not lecture to parents.
3. Use simple language with examples and illustrations.
4. Direct the parents toward steps they can take. This allows them quickly to feel a part of the intervention process.
5. Say what must be said pleasantly but bluntly in response to questions. Do not hedge on what must be said on the assumption that the parents may reject it.
6. Recall that you may be relating information to the parents that they have feared hearing for some time.

The assessor should be prepared to deal with a wide variety of questions the parents may pose. These may relate to the cause of the developmental delay noted, the degree of the delay present, what the future holds, further treatment or intervention for the delay, and issues that relate to family adjustment to the needs engendered by having a special child.

Goal Three: Providing Release and Support

As a part of the intake interview, the assessor must be alert to the need of parents to express frustrations, fears, and anger. These emotions may relate to a variety of causes. For the most part, however, they usually relate to the parents' attempt to adjust and deal with the responsibilities of having a developmentally delayed child. An array of potentially confusing choices face the parents. They may need assistance in understanding and in making the best choice for their child. They may need encouragement about their ability to meet their child's needs. The interviewer must be prepared to handle these emotions. Should the interviewer sense that the parents may experience difficulty, then additional professional assistance may be sought. In general, the assessor is in a better position to gain a complete picture of developmental performance if the parents are given full opportunity to express themselves. It is the rare set of parents who will not communicate honestly with the assessor once a genuine caring attitude is sensed.

DEVELOPMENTAL SCREENING

Many infant-toddler practitioners are involved in activities that are primarily screening in nature. One major goal of developmental screening is to identify children, during their infant and toddler years, who appear to be asymptomatic but who are likely to develop a developmental deficit that interferes with the expected sequence of normal growth and development. Screening has been defined as the "presumptive identification of unrecognized disease or defects by the application of tests, examinations, or other procedures which can be applied rapidly" (Kemper and Frankenburg, 1979, p. 12). During a screening, a binary decision is reached on whether a particular child is developing with or without problems. Table 5-1 presents a list of sample screening instruments and the domains covered by each.

TABLE 5-1. Examples of selected screening instruments

Test	Administration time (min)	Age range	Domains covered
Receptive-Expressive Emergent Language Scale	20	0–3 months	Language
Denver Developmental Screening Test	20	0–5 years	Global
Home Observation for Measurement in the Environment	60 per section	0–5 years	Parent-child interaction
Infant Intelligence Scale	30	0–3 years	Cognition
Minnesota Infant Development Inventory	30	0–2 years	Global

Children who are identified as having abnormal screening results are referred for a more complete neurodevelopmental evaluation. In theory, all infants and toddlers should receive some degree of formal or informal screening as part of regular monitoring of their growth and development. In actual practice, however, this is not the case. Shonkoff, Dworkin, and Leviton (1979) reported that only 25 percent of pediatricians use any type of formal developmental screening tool. Most pediatricians rely solely on their subjective clinical judgment to determine whether an infant or toddler displays a normal pattern of developmental skill acquisition.

Coplan (1982) measured pediatricians' ability to judge accurately cognitive performance in their patients. In several studies designed to compare physicians' subjective estimate of intelligence quotient (IQ) with actual developmental-cognitive scores, the correlations ranged from .32 to .65. The tendency was to lump all patients toward the middle of the distribution curve, cutting off both the upper and lower ends. An additional study designed to determine how developmentally delayed children's problems were identified and how the medical system was involved has been conducted by Palfrey, Singer, Walker, and Butler (1987). The developmental problems that were investigated include speech problems, learning disabilities, emotional disturbance, mental retardation, sensory disorders, and physical health disabilities. Overall, 4.5 percent of the children's problems were identified at birth and only 28.7 percent before the age of 5 years.

The authors conclude that a better systematic sharing of responsibility for the early identification of developmentally disabling conditions is needed. They further stated that pediatricians should, at the very least, devote a half-hour visit to the developmental assessment of each child in the 3- to 5-year age range. What these studies reveal is that routine screening of developmental skill acquisition does not appear to be taking place as much as it should, at least within the medical community.

A variety of methods can be used to screen the developmental progress of infants and toddlers. These methods may include the administration of formal screening instruments such as the *Denver Developmental Screening Test* (DDST) (Frankenburg, Dodds, Fandal, Kazuk, and Cohrs, 1975). The DDST is designed to help the health provider detect developmental pathology. Widely used by a variety of professionals as a valuable tool in early identification of potential developmental delay, it requires administration by a trained examiner. Items on the DDST are arranged in four sections: personal-social development, fine motor-adaptive development, language development, and gross motor development. A child may be tested multiple times from birth through age 6 using the same instrument.

The items on the DDST were selected from more than 12 developmental and preschool intelligence tests. They were chosen based on their ease of administration and clarity in scoring. Available normative data allow the assessor to compare obtained performance with developmental norms to assist in determining a particular child's developmental status. In general the DDST represents a more structured and formal manner of screening developmental skill mastery.

A less formal methodology for screening developmental skill acquisition may include short checklists of developmental behaviors that parents or others can use as a basis for comparison. These checklists may be formal or relatively informal. The items covered may include developmental milestones that represent all modalities or may be domain specific. Screening of this nature can be completed by parents or other persons with access to the child. It is not uncommon to see checklists regarding development in newspaper articles, physicians' offices, or other public places. Screening devices of this nature usually contain information regarding who to contact should parents have concerns about their child's development. Figure 5-2 outlines a sample screening device used to gauge speech and language development.

Figure 5-2. Screening instrument: Birth to three years of age. (Adapted from the University of Illinois Parents of Infants and Young Children Materials, Department of Speech and Hearing Science, Champaign, Illinois.)

CHILD'S AGE (MO)	BEHAVIOR	ANSWER	
0–6	Does child turn to sound?	Yes	No
	Does child smile when talked to?	Yes	No
	Does child make sounds when talked to?	Yes	No
6–12	Does child respond to name?	Yes	No
	Does child understand "no-no"?	Yes	No
	Does child "babble"?	Yes	No
12–18	Does child respond to simple instructions?	Yes	No
	Does child respond to simple yes and no questions?	Yes	No
	Can child say more than three words?	Yes	No
24–36	Can child identify objects by their use?	Yes	No
	Does child use pronouns (I, me, you)?	Yes	No
	Does child ask questions and lead you in simple conversation?	Yes	No

If you have answered "no" to any of these questions in your child's age group, your child may have a speech, language, or hearing disorder. To find out more about your child's speech and language development, contact _____ .

A secondary benefit to the use of developmental screening activities is that parents find it helpful to know that children vary in their patterns of individual developmental growth. Whether it is during the newborn period, infancy, or preschool period, parents appreciate reassurance about the status of their child's development. Parents benefit from familiarity with the concept that developmental progress is characterized by unevenness, irregularities, and starts and stops. Hence, developmental screening not only assists in the early detection of developmental pathology, but also provides an optimal opportunity for the caregiver to become acquainted with various aspects of overall infant-toddler development.

The overall principle that governs screening activity is that it is an opportunity for the assessor to observe or become aware of various samples of infant-toddler behavior and to make a preliminary judgment regarding the appropriateness of the observed-reported behavior. If the behavior is considered to be age appropriate, then the child might be scheduled for an additional screening within a specified time (6 or 12 months). If the child displays behavior that causes the assessor to question either the child's age appropriateness of current behavior or potential for future developmental progress, then additional referrals for more detailed developmental assessment can be initiated. Developmental screening is not designed to provide detailed descriptions or samples of developmental performance. Rather, it is designed to provide a basis of information regarding developmental progress on which to make judgments about the need for more in-depth assessment.

TYPES OF ASSESSMENT INSTRUMENTS

A concept frequently used in consideration of the process of assessment is that the assessor is involved in diagnostic activity. In many instances the word *diagnosis* is applied to infant assessment. The use of this word is best left in the medical model, however, because a medical diagnosis leads to definitive statements about etiology, clinical symptomatology, treatment, and prognosis. In sharp contrast, educational or psychological testing provides little if any information about etiology, some but not much about clinical symptomatology, and absolutely none about prognosis. A single test permits some decisions about the presence or absence of some clinical conditions, but, as has been previously stated, the younger the child, the less reliable these observations. A single test administration can be viewed as only a glimpse into child behavior on a particular day and under a particular set of circumstances. This must be kept in mind when choosing actual assessment instruments.

GLOBAL ASSESSMENT INSTRUMENTS

An additional consideration that must be addressed in choosing assessment instruments relates to the general type of outcome the assessor desires. There are advantages as well as disadvantages in the use of test procedures that yield a global score resulting in a developmental quotient. For example, several instruments are designed to assess a variety of areas related to overall development. Test instruments that fit under this category include the *Bayley Scales of Infant Development* or the *McCarthy Scale of Children's Abilities* (Bayley, 1969; McCarthy, 1972). Although each of these instruments assesses various modalities as part of the test protocol, each yields a global summary score that can be expressed as a raw score, an age equivalency score, a developmental quotient, or a developmental IQ. The McCarthy scale provides a breakdown of performance in each of the areas that constitutes the test. In addition, a score reflecting the combination of all scores is also available.

Tests of this nature are usually comprehensive and possess strong reliability and validity. Tests that provide global information regarding performance, although powerful tools, must be used by the assessor with certain factors in mind. The global score obtained reflects developmental performance across all modalities. In other words, the score obtained indicates the summary of how a particular child did in total and not within specific domains. Various instruments permit a domain-by-domain review of results; the global score is the compilation of performance across domains.

The basic premise underlying global scores is that all areas assessed reflect general developmental skill mastery equally. In essence, every skill is weighed equally, and as such all areas assessed can contribute positively or negatively to the global score obtained. Given the comprehensive nature of instruments of this type, it is not surprising that the administrator must possess familiarity with the instrument, preferably through adequate training and practice.

The main concern in obtaining a global score in the manner specified above is that the exact relationship between mastery or lack of mastery in specific areas and the total score obtained is simply not known. For example, a global score may be reduced because of delay in the motor domain. This may indicate a concurrent developmental delay in the sociocommunicative domain. The skilled assessor must always bear in mind inherent limitations and cautions in using global scores and in comparing those scores with normative data. The result may be that a particular child is judged to be at a performance level that does not truly reflect developmental skills.

DOMAIN-SPECIFIC ASSESSMENT INSTRUMENTS

In contrast to the types of instruments specified above, the outcome of domain-specific instruments does not reflect global overall developmental skill status but rather the developmental level of a specific developmental domain. Practitioners from across disciplines are familiar with assessment instruments authored by colleagues in each discipline that are designed to assess a specific skill area. Tests of this nature are not designed to, nor do they attempt to, provide assessment data apart from that which relate to a specific area of development. Appendix B gives numerous examples of domain-specific assessment instruments. In essence, domain-specific instruments zero in on one area of development. For example, the *Assessing Prelinguistic and Linguistic Behaviors in Developmentally Young Children* assessment tool (Olswang, Stoel Gammons, Coggins, and Carpenter, 1987) is designed to assess the prelinguistic and early linguistic behaviors of infants and toddlers. It does not attempt to assess motor functioning, nor does it address issues related to the home environment or child-caregiver relationship (outside of the play context). It breaks down prelinguistic and linguistic behaviors into five categories all related to preverbal and verbal areas of functioning: cognitive antecedents to word meaning, play scale, communicative intention scale, language comprehension scale, and language production scale. Numerous examples exist of instruments that assess language skills, motor development, cognitive development, and issues related to family functioning. The assessor must keep these broad categories of instruments in mind when deciding which specific instrument or type of test to use when assessment activity is initiated. The following chapter, in a discussion of specific test procedures, provides further information regarding the application of specific tests, both domain specific and global.

NORM-REFERENCED ASSESSMENT INSTRUMENTS

In general, two broad categories of infant-toddler assessment instruments are used with greatest frequency. These are norm- and criterion-referenced tests. A norm-referenced test is one that affords the assessor the opportunity to discriminate among the performance of a group of people and thus interpret how an individual's performance compares with that of the group. In essence, a norm-referenced test allows the assessor to view an individual's performance with reference to group performance on similar tasks. The data obtained on norm-referenced instruments may be obtained through direct testing of the child, through observation of child behaviors, or in some instances through parental, caregiver, and possibly teacher interview data.

The outcome of norm-referenced tests may be reflected in the establishment of developmental ages, developmental quotients, perceptual quotients, age level scores, mental age or IQ scores, general scale indexes, or overall profiles of global performance. Often, percentile scores are derived from test results. Thus, the examiner is able to indicate that a particular infant or toddler compares in a favorable or unfavorable manner with other infants or toddlers. It is apparent that there is inherent value in obtaining assessment results that afford this type of performance review. It is just as important that the assessor keep in mind some of the limitations outlined previously about global results on assessment instruments. Many of the same cautions exist. Table 5-2 presents a selected sample of norm-referenced assessment instruments.

TABLE 5-2. Selected norm-referenced assessment instruments

Test	*Domains covered*	*Outcomes*
Kent Infant Development Scale	Cognitive Motor Social Language Self-help	Developmental age and profile of skills
Bayley Scales of Infant Development	Mental Psychomotor	Developmental quotient Developmental age
Gesell Developmental Schedules	Communication Gross motor Fine motor Adaptive Personal-social	Developmental quotient Maturity age
Peabody Picture Vocabulary Test	Receptive language	Age level
Sequenced Inventory of Communication Development	Receptive and expressive communication	Age level
Stanford–Binet Intelligence Scale	General intelligence	Mental age, IQ
McCarthy Scale of Children's Abilities	Verbal Perceptual Quantitative Cognitive Memory Motor	Scale index General cognitive index

Source: Adapted from D. Bricker (1986). Early education of at risk and handicapped infants, toddlers, and preschool children. Glenview, IL: Scott, Foresman and Company.

CRITERION-REFERENCED ASSESSMENT INSTRUMENTS

The second prominent category of infant-toddler assessment instruments is known as criterion-referenced tests. Criterion-referenced tests are those in which content is defined in terms of some specific performance dimension or interest. Criterion-referenced assessment instruments assess the performance of an individual relative to a well-defined behavioral domain and indicate mastery or nonmastery of that particular item. In essence, criterion-referenced measures provide an overall indication of pass-fail performance on a well-defined aspect of behavior.

Administration procedures are not as strictly standardized as those for norm-referenced tests. The actual administration procedures may include direct testing of the child or interview data gathered from persons in a position to provide accurate data regarding behaviors the child displays. Instruments of this nature do not yield age norm data, although some do provide "age equivalence" information for each item or level on the instrument. The cumulative pass-fail indicators aid the assessor in determining the appropriateness of a particular child's developmental level.

The overall purpose of measures of this nature is to determine whether the individual's performance demonstrates mastery over the behaviors under observation. Based on the responses elicited, an individual's behavior is judged to be proficient or nonproficient. The results may be tied to specific curricular suggestions and may in essence provide a direct basis for intervention goals and objectives. After data are collected on all the items that constitute the criterion-referenced instrument, an overall percentage of pass-fail can be computed. Based on this percentage, judgments regarding overall mastery can be formed. For example, mastery of 85 percent of the items might be considered sufficient for success. Percentages of mastery that are considered success may vary from age to age. Thus, an individual child's performance of specific behaviors can be compared with another child's behavior or to group behavior in determining mastery of the target behavior. Tables 5-3 and 5-4 show a breakdown of several assessment instruments and whether they are norm- or criterion-referenced and global or domain specific. Table 5-5 presents a sample of criterion-referenced infant-toddler assessment instruments.

DEVELOPMENTAL LOG

One additional comment about types of assessment information concerns an expansion of what was previously mentioned in reference to parental data. Parents are a primary source of valuable data concerning their child's developmental progress. Data kept by parents over time, which describes in chronologic order the development of new skills, can be a rich source of

TABLE 5-3. Norm- and criterion-referenced global assessment instruments

Norm referenced	Criterion referenced
McCarthy Scale of Children's Abilities	Memphis Comprehensive Development Scale
Bayley Scales of Infant Development	
Kent Infant Development Scale	Uniform Performance Assessment System
Minnesota Child Development Inventory	Early Intervention Development Profile
	Adaptive Performance Instrument
	Denver Developmental Screening Test

TABLE 5-4. Norm- and criterion-referenced domain-specific assessment instruments

Norm referenced	Criterion referenced
Peabody Picture Vocabulary Test	Assessing Linguistic Behaviors
Receptive Expressive Emergent Language Scale	Early Language Milestones
	Boyd Developmental Progress Scale
Test of Early Socio-Emotional Development	Vineland Social Maturity Scale
Developmental Test of Visual-Motor Integration	Environmental Pre-Language Battery
Early Language Inventory	Milani–Comparetti Developmental Scale

information for the assessor. Data of this nature can certainly assist in the selection of assessment instruments. They can also be used in instances where standard test instruments are not applicable for a particular child due to sensory impairment or other reasons.

Another use for data of this nature deals with how parental reporting that covers child change over time coincides with the results on formal assessment activity. Hence, the use of a developmental log is advised. There need not be any set structure or format to the log; however, the assessor may find it helpful to provide parents with some guidance for log maintenance. Parents have proved to be proficient describers of behavior, and it would be a waste not to consider, and in some instances weigh equally, their data on the child's skill progress. Parents can be instructed to chart new skills as

TABLE 5-5. Selected criterion-referenced assessment instruments

Test	Domains covered	Outcomes
Brigance Diagnostic Inventory of Early Development	Motor Speech-language Preacademic	Performance level and developmental age level
Hawaii Early Learning Profile (HELP)	Cognitive Language Gross motor Fine motor Social-emotional Self-help	Profile of skill level; approximate age levels
Home Observation for Measurement of the Environment (HOME Inventory)	Home environment	Inventory of support available to the child in the home
Memphis Comprehensive Development Scale (MCDS)	Personal-social Gross motor Fine motor Language Perceptocognitive	Profile for individual programming
Uniform Performance Assessment System (UPAS)	Preacademic Fine motor Communication Social self-help Gross motor Behavior	Profile of skill level

Source: Adapted from D. Bricker (1986). Early education of at risk and handicapped infants, toddlers, and preschool children. Glenview, IL: Scott, Foresman and Company.

the child learns them. The parents can be directed simply to note the date and briefly describe the new skill learned. Great detail is not necessary. Rather, the value of a log lies in the descriptions of change seen over time. These descriptions can assist the examiner in actual test selection. More important, though, they can provide the basis on which to make judgments regarding developmental adequacy in the absence of formal test administration.

INTERPRETATION OF RESULTS

Regardless of the type of assessment instrument employed, a general philosophy of test results interpretation must be available to the assessor. Included in this philosophy should be an understanding of how the results will be used as the child's future needs are considered. Once all data regarding the child have been collected, either from a single test administration or as the result of serial assessment, a decision must be made about the child's performance adequacy. The assessment results are crucial, since a host of decisions hinge on them. These decisions relate to the need for additional medical intervention and early intervention, the effectiveness of current intervention, school placement, and strengths and weaknesses within individual developmental domains.

In general, assessment results can be viewed as either prognostic or prescriptive. A combination of the two is also possible. A prognostic interpretation of assessment results is one in which the assessor makes long-term predictions on future potential, needs, and expectations based on the results of a single test administration. A prognostic interpretation of assessment results is, in almost all instances, tenuous. This is, however, lessened somewhat if the child has been evaluated several times over time. Nevertheless, even in the presence of serial observations, the assessor must be cautious in making long-term prognostic assumptions based on child performance. Previous discussions have centered on the lack of predictive ability of current infant-toddler assessment instruments. There are too many variables related to the child and the environment to make prognostic statements reliable.

In general, the younger the child and the fewer the observational opportunities, the less correlation there is between early assessment results and later performance in the absence of severe neurologic damage or known mental retardation syndromes. As the child's age increases, and as additional assessments are performed over time, the prognostic benefit of assessment increases somewhat but is by no means foolproof. The assessor is cautioned, therefore, about making long-term judgments about a child's developmental potential on the basis of results obtained early in the child's life or on the basis of a limited sample of behaviors.

A second and more helpful manner in which to view assessment results is to view them in a prescriptive manner. This is simply to answer the question, "What is the next step of action based on what has been obtained?" A prescriptive approach toward viewing assessment results can result in a variety of outcomes. For an infant seen at an early age who performs below expectations, the decision may simply be to ask the parents to keep a developmental log and to schedule the child for reassessment in 90 days. If a persistent pattern of developmental delay is present over six to nine months, the decision may be to provide the parents with instruction and home stimulation materials to initiate intervention in the home setting.

It is also likely that a child who displays a persistent pattern of development delay will be referred to an early intervention program for potential home- or center-based intervention activities. If the child is already involved in intervention activities, a prescriptive view of assessment results may focus on specific developmental domains to direct intervention efforts in a more concentrated manner in these areas. A prescriptive view of assessment results also requires the assessor to be alert to additional referrals that may be needed. These may include the need for additional medical evaluation and intervention or the need to see other members of the interdisciplinary team. In short, a prescriptive use of assessment results requires the assessor to look ahead to the next step of action for the child. The choices range from no action to intense intervention and further assessment.

COMMUNICATION OF ASSESSMENT RESULTS

In one form or another, assessment results, once obtained by the assessor, must be communicated to a variety of persons interested in child development issues. It is imperative that the infant-toddler assessor keep in mind the particular audience to which assessment results will be disseminated. By so doing, both confusion and ineffectiveness can be avoided when communicating results with parents and other professionals.

COMMUNICATION WITH PARENTS

Previous discussion made a distinction between the basic types of interviews that the assessor might conduct with parents. The intake (direct) interview is designed to acquire as much relevant information as possible before the actual assessment. These data assist the assessor in better understanding the samples of behavior that will be obtained. Data of this nature also assist the assessor in selecting appropriate test instruments, since an initial familiarity with the unique aspects of a particular child are of interest as decisions regarding appropriate instruments are made.

Following the actual assessment, the data that are transmitted to parents must be precise and clear and must be presented in a manner that allows the parents the opportunity to understand assessment results fully. The assessor must keep in mind the emotional stake the parents may have in the results obtained. In some instances, and this should not be underestimated, the infant-toddler assessor is the first professional to indicate to the parents that their child may not be functioning normally. This is no light matter and should be taken quite seriously by the assessor. One hopes that these instances are the exception rather than the norm.

If the assessor suspects that the parents will have a difficult time adjusting to the information shared regarding child performance, care must be taken to present information in an empathetic and compassionate manner. Sufficient time must be allowed for the parents to adapt to the presence of a delay in their child. It may be necessary for the assessor to suggest that the parents see other members of the interdisciplinary team in an effort to enhance parental acceptance and adjustment to the changes inherent in meeting the needs of a handicapped infant or toddler. Decisions must be made on an individual basis by the assessor in such instances. Experience is the best teacher regarding the assessor's ability to read the situation and act appropriately.

On the other hand, many parents have suspected for some time that their child is not developing normally. They may have seen a number of medical and developmental specialists and are familiar with many aspects of the developmental pathology present in their child. In those instances where the parents suspected a problem, the assessor may choose to inform parents that assessment results confirm the presence of a delay and then continue to describe the nature of the delay in greater detail. Once parents sense that the assessor has the child's best interest in mind and that all questions they have will be addressed by the assessor, the tendency is to turn attention more toward what can be done rather than toward where the "fault" lies. Recall that assessment results are better viewed from the "What next?" framework. Parents can be quickly directed toward future steps that should be taken regardless of whether the action suggested is assessment or intervention.

In many instances, the samples of behavior noted may indicate that the infant or toddler is functioning near age expectations in all developmental domains. If assessment results point in that direction, then the recommendations might simply be to reassess the child in six months as a final gauge of developmental adequacy. In the case of the infant who is demonstrating a moderate-to-severe degree of a developmental pathology, and who has been seen over time by the assessor, the parents are in most instances quite familiar with the unique needs their child has. Discussions in these instances should be sensitive but directed ultimately toward subsequent courses of action based on current assessment results (answering the "What next?" question). In any case, the assessor must be prepared to deal with all possible questions parents may have as well as all possible responses regarding what the assessor is communicating to them about their child.

COMMUNICATION WITH OTHER PROFESSIONALS

Communication with other professionals should also be with the intended audience in mind. Clear descriptions of the tests used, the child's performance, and test interpretation should be provided. If the test used provides a variety of ways to describe performance (e.g., percentile data, developmental age), these should also be indicated. Remember, however, that not all practitioners are familiar with the variety of assessment tools available. If the assessor is assessing a specific skill area, professionals from other disciplines may not be familiar with the specific instrument used. In such instances, a brief description of the test employed should prove helpful to the person receiving assessment results. The overall interpretation of the performance obtained should be transmitted clearly and in a manner that is easy to comprehend. In those instances when an accurate interpretation of behaviors observed is impossible, the assessor should simply describe observed behaviors. Clear descriptions and reports of results will enhance services provided to an infant or toddler as well as allow persons from other disciplines to feel a part of the total effort directed toward the child.

SUMMARY

If assessment is viewed as a data-collection technique, then the assessor's goal is to collect as reliable and accurate a sample of data as possible. The present chapter has pointed out that a variety of data-collection techniques are available to the assessor. These include case history, questionnaire, interview, developmental log, and direct testing of the child. The accuracy of the data collected depends in large measure on the assessor's expertise, regardless of the specific technique chosen. Important decisions regarding future courses of action for the infant and toddler hinge on the collection of accurate and reliable samples of behavior. The experienced assessor realizes that infant-toddler assessment is more than simply administering a test. Data from all sources must be treated with respect and included in the decision-making process.

STUDY QUESTIONS

1. What is the difference between the direct (intake) and the interpretative interview? What purposes does each fulfill? What areas might the assessor want to cover in each?
2. Several broad categories of assessment instruments were discussed in this chapter. What are these? What factors should the assessor keep in mind when selecting assessment instruments?
3. What is a developmental log? How might a log be of assistance to the assessor?
4. Communicating assessment results with parents and other professionals must be taken quite seriously. What factors should the assessor keep in mind as results are communicated to various people?

REFERENCES

Bayley, N. (1969). *Bayley scales of infant development.* New York: The Psychological Corporation.

Bricker, D. (1986). *Early education of at risk and handicapped infants, toddlers, and preschool children.* Glenview, IL: Scott, Foresman and Company.

Coplan, J. (1982). Parental estimate of child's developmental level in a high risk population. *American Journal of Disorders in Childhood, 136,* 101.

Emerick, L. (1969). *The parent interview.* Danville, IL: Interstate Printers.

Frankenburg, W., Dodds, J., Fandal, A., Kazuk, E., & Cohrs, M. (1975). *Denver Developmental Screening Test: Reference manual.* Boulder, CO: University of Colorado Medical Center.

Kemper, M., & Frankenburg, W. (1979). Screening, diagnosis, and assessment: How do these types of measurments differ? In T. Black (Ed.), *Perspectives on measurement: A collection of readings for educators of young handicapped children.* Chapel Hill: Technical Assistance Development System.

McCarthy, D. (1972). *McCarthy scales of children's abilities.* Chicago: The Psychological Corporation.

Palfrey, J., Singer, J., Walker, D., & Butler, J. (1987). Early identification of children's special needs: A study of 5 metropolitan communities. *Journal of Pediatrics, 11,* 651.

Shonkoff, J., Dworkin, P., & Leviton, A. (1979). Primary case approaches to developmental disabilities. *Pediatrics, 64,* 506.

CHAPTER 6

Specific Assessment Domains and Procedures

Specific Developmental
Domains to be Assessed
   Language Domain
   Motor Domain
   Cognitive Domain
   Family Assessment

Summary

Study Questions

References

Assessment activity directed toward infants and toddlers is a complex process that consists of posing and effectively answering a variety of questions that arise concerning the child's developmental adequacy. These questions relate primarily to the nature of the child's behavior and focus on the child's abilities or disabilities. Assessment is central to the spectrum of services provided for infants and toddlers. It must always be viewed as an ongoing process. Practitioners, regardless of discipline, must have a common philosophy and goal in mind for the outcome of their services.

No shortage of information exists on specific assessment activities within any number of developmental areas. The complex nature of assessment, even within a single developmental domain, can overwhelm the practitioner. This feeling of being overwhelmed can be even greater if a single practitioner attempts to become adept at assessment activity that crosses his or her primary discipline. It is with the full realization of the difficulty of displaying assessment proficiency across developmental domains that the present chapter is undertaken.

The material to follow is not intended to provide in-depth coverage of assessment within each developmental domain. Rather, it is designed to help the practitioner better understand the unique aspects of assessment outside of his or her primary academic discipline. Issues regarding the positive or negative aspects of the various assessment instruments referred to in this chapter are not discussed (Appendix B provides an exhaustive listing of assessment instruments across developmental domains). It is the distinct purpose of this chapter to teach the practitioner that infant-toddler assessment is not a cookbook process in which a prescribed set of rules are followed. Rather, assessment is a process through which reliable samples of infant-toddler behavior are obtained. Some behaviors are obtained in a highly structured manner; others are obtained in a less stringent fashion. All behaviors are used in making inferences about the child's developmental level. It is ultimately the assessor's responsibility to select the methods that best accomplish this purpose.

SPECIFIC DEVELOPMENTAL DOMAINS TO BE ASSESSED

LANGUAGE DOMAIN

With advancing knowledge about infant communication, practitioners are now more aware of the importance of early identification and remediation for communication disorders. Increased data on the importance of early communicative opportunity between the infant and the primary caregiver stimulated interest in strategies to gauge the quantity and quality of caregiver-infant interaction. Hence, more assessment tools aimed specifically at infant-caregiver interaction have appeared. In addition, new tools to assess a variety of areas related to infant-toddler communicative effectiveness have emerged. Many of these tools are mentioned in the material to follow. The first area within the language domain to be discussed is that of infant-caregiver interaction.

Infant-Caregiver Interaction

Interaction cues and responses of normal newborns include eye contact, crying, quieting, attention to faces and voices, and body movements. Infant-caregiver interactions that are in synchrony are thought to have long-term effects on cognitive, social, and linguistic skills (Sparks, Clark, Das, and Erickson, 1988). The fact that many infants are not afforded an optimal opportunity to establish a stable relationship with a primary caregiver is well established. Take, for example, the child who spends four to ten weeks in an intensive care nursery. During much of that time the infant may be in an inturned state (see Chapter 4). Thus, the child is directing all physiologic energy toward survival. There is simply no energy to spare for establishing a reciprocal relationship with a caregiver.

In addition, substantial stress is placed on the mother as she must adjust to the fact that her child is ill and will not be coming home as soon as she would like. The amount of time that the mother is able to spend with the child is related directly to the quality of interaction between them. Tables 6-1 and 6-2 present data on the mean number of days and the amount of rehospitalization required of premature infants. This information serves to

TABLE 6-1. Mean days in the neonatal intensive care nursery for surviving infants by birth weight

Birth weight status (gm)	Days in nursery
Above 2,500	3.5
2,001–2,500	7.0
1,501–2,000	24.0
Below 1,500	57.0
Below 1,000	89.0

Source: Adapted from Committee to Study the Prevention of Low Birth Weight (1985). *Preventing low birth weight*. Washington, DC: Institute of Medicine.

**TABLE 6-2. Rehospitalization of babies
in their first year by birth weight**

Birth weight status (gm)	Hospitalized (%)	Length of stay (days)
Below 1,500	40	16
Below 2,500	19	12.5
Above 2,500	8.7	8.9

Source: Adapted from Committee to Study the Prevention of Low Birth Weight (1985). *Preventing low
birth weight.* Washington, DC: Institute of Medicine.

amplify further the difficulty in establishing an optimal mother-infant interactional pattern in the early days of life.

As an additional means of underscoring the lack of interactional opportunity afforded the child while in the hospital, High and Gorski (1985)
monitored the amount and type of caregiver interaction between medical
personnel and infants. Their data quantified the interactions seen between
medical personnel and infants while the babies were in the intensive care
nursery. Both acutely ill and convalescing infants were observed. A summary of the results revealed the following.

1. *Percentage of time nurse was present.* Nurses were present for
   only 30 percent of the acute observations and 20 percent of the
   convalescent observations.
2. *Percentage of time no caregiver was present.* No caregiver of any
   kind was present for 63 percent of the acute observation periods
   and 71 percent of the convalescent ones. These statistics may reflect staffing patterns that assign one nurse to several infants when
   they no longer require critical care.
3. *Interval between nurse completing a caregiving task and leaving
   the infant's care area.* Nurses spent 85 seconds for acute and 64
   seconds for convalescent groups from completing an intervention
   to leaving the infant's care area.
4. *Amount and type of handling.* Thirteen percent of total observation time included some form of caregiver touching of infants. For
   acute observations, most touching involved medical procedures
   (71%), while a nearly equal amount of medical and social touching
   (54% versus 60%) was experienced by convalescent infants.

The results of the High and Gorski investigation underscore the reality that
less-than-optimal interaction patterns are seen as part of the normal nur-

sery routine. Note that these patterns of interaction can exist in the presence of high-quality medical care.

The importance of early mother-infant interactions was further emphasized in an investigation by Jacobson, Starnes, and Gasser (1988). These authors pointed out that mothers who do not talk frequently to their premature babies generally have infants who score lower on developmental scales than do mothers who provide frequent language stimulation. The study reviewed the effectiveness of an in-hospital training program designed to increase mothers' production of descriptions and praises directed to their infants. Mothers with low baseline rates of talking to their premature infants were trained to produce descriptions and praises. Results indicated that mothers significantly increased their frequency of descriptions and praises and that these skills remained strong one month after training ended. Innovative research of this nature underscores the importance of early mother-infant interaction. Hence, the value of early detection of interaction deficiencies is fully realized.

In an attempt to identify deficient mother-infant interaction (communication) patterns, Klein and Briggs (1986) devised a scale that may be used in observing the communicative interaction present between mother and infant. The authors indicate that the *Observation of Communicative Interaction* (OCI) was developed for use as an informal observation guide to assist program staff in describing the interaction strategies used by parents. The authors further indicate that the OCI is intended as a clinical observation tool. It should be used as an informal guide to qualitative assessment of relative strengths and weaknesses of caregiver-infant interaction. It is not designed as a research instrument. There are no data on the instrument's reliability or validity. The data collected as part of the OCI can be used to monitor progress and change over time. The ratings provided on the OCI can help identify relative strengths and weaknesses in caregivers' interaction patterns and provide guidance for planning individual target goals, intervention strategies, and interaction activities.

The OCI may be administered during an observation in which the caregiver is engaged in a routine interaction with the infant. It outlines ten interaction categories around which observations are targeted. Figure 6-1 presents an adapted scoring form based on the OCI. No specific age guidelines are provided with the OCI. It is also structured to yield valuable information regarding the quality and style of mother-infant interaction. Interactional pathology detected at an early age is more amenable to treatment and intervention. If they are left untreated, communicative pathology is more likely to occur at a later date.

An additional approach toward monitoring the type of interaction present between mother and infant is provided by Seibert and Hogan (1982). These authors devised the *Early Social Communication Scales* (ESCS), which is designed to gauge the type and quality of interaction between infant and

ITEM	RARELY/NEVER	SOMETIMES	OFTEN
1. Provides appropriate tactile and kinesthetic stimulation (strokes, pats, caresses, cuddles, and rocks baby).	☐	☐	☐
2. Mother displays pleasure while interacting with baby.	☐	☐	☐
3. Mother responds to child's distress.	☐	☐	☐
4. Positions self and infant so eye-to-eye contact is possible (facing and 7–12 inches away).	☐	☐	☐
5. Smiles contingently at infant.	☐	☐	☐
6. Varies prosodic features (higher pitch, talks slower, exaggerated intonation).	☐	☐	☐
7. Encourages conversation.	☐	☐	☐
8. Responds contingently to infant's behavior.	☐	☐	☐
9. Modifies interaction in response to negative cues from infant.	☐	☐	☐
10. Uses communication to teach language and concepts.	☐	☐	☐

Figure 6-1. Observation of communicative interaction scoring sheet (OCI). (Adapted from D. Klein and M. Briggs [1986]. Observation of communicative interaction. A model program to facilitate positive communication interactions between caregivers and their high risk infants [DHHS Publication No. MCJ 06351-01-0]. Washington, DC: Government Printing Office.

caregiver. Table 6-3 presents a sample of the social dimensions assessed as part of the ESCS.

The items outlined in Table 6-3 are designed to serve as a barometer for the degree to which the infant seeks out, responds to, or initiates social interaction. It has been established that the infant, at least in the early stages of interaction, sets the overall tone of the interaction. Hence, as the infant is better able to interact with caregivers, the amount, type, and style

**TABLE 6-3. Early social
communication scale
dimensions**

SOCIAL INTERACTION

Child responds to
Child initiates
Child maintains

JOINT ATTENTION

Child responds to
Child initiates
Child maintains

BEHAVIOR REGULATION

Child responds to
Child initiates
Child maintains

Source: Adapted from J. Seibert
and A. Hogan (1982). A model
for assessing social and object
skills and planning intervention.
In D. McClowery (Ed.), *Infant
Communication Development:
Assessment and Intervention.*
New York: Grune & Stratton.

of interaction between mother and infant becomes richer and more complex. These interactions serve as precursors to more complex forms of
communication that will develop later.

A specific instrument designed for use in rating live or videotaped interactions of mothers and infants four to six weeks after birth is the *Mother-
Infant Play Interaction Scale* (MIPIS). Walker and Thompson (1982)
describe the scale as being designed to rate a five-minute session of unstructured play in the home setting. The MIPIS was developed to measure
strategies that mothers use to elicit social behavior from their infants and,
in turn, infant responsiveness to these attempts at socialization. Mothers are
instructed to play with their infants for five minutes doing the kinds of
things they would normally do with them when not feeding, bathing, or
changing them. No constraints are placed on the mother in regard to placing the infant or the particular interactive strategies. The main point is to
preserve the ecologic validity of the interaction session. Table 6-4 shows
the 16 areas that the MIPIS rates on a five-point scale.

A cautionary note regarding the assessment of parent-child interactions
must be added at this point: It is difficult to quantify the nature of parent-
child interaction. Although certain behaviors have been alluded to in the

TABLE 6-4. **Mother-infant play interaction scale items**

1. Maternal holding style
2. Maternal expression of affect
3. Maternal expression of affect — quality of contingency to infant
4. Maternal caregiving style
5. Predominant infant wakeful response level
6. Predominant infant mood and affect
7. Maternal visual interaction
8. Infant visual interaction
9. Style of play — animate versus inanimate interaction
10. Maternal vocalization style — general (tone and content)
11. Maternal vocalization style — quantity of contingency
12. Maternal attempts at smile elicitation
13. Kinesthetic quality of interaction
14. Overall didactic quality of interaction
15. Synchrony of affect
16. Termination of interaction

Source: Adapted from L. Walker and E. Thompson (1982). Mother-infant play interaction scale. In S. Humenic–Smith (Ed.), *Analysis of current assessment in the health care of young children and childbearing families.* Norwich, CT: Appleton-Century-Crofts.

instruments identified above, it is quite difficult to attach a weighted value to behaviors that are assumed to reflect optimal parent-child interaction. Interaction patterns may vary widely from family to family as well as from culture to culture. Although the exact nature of the interactions may show variation, these same interactions may be equally nurturing. In addition, even if deficient patterns are suspected, should the behaviors that are not observed (based on the administration of a particular instrument) be those targeted in intervention? Clearly, more research is needed on what creates optimal levels of parent-child interaction.

Maternal Attachment

The issue of maternal attachment is an important one, especially as it relates to establishing optimal mother-infant interactional patterns. If various factors in the child's early experience make the establishment of attachment tenuous, then it can be said that the development of optimal interactional patterns are also at risk.

Attachment can be defined as a unique relationship between two people that lasts over time (Klaus and Kennell, 1976). Although quantifying attachment during the early periods of the infant's life can be difficult, behaviors such as fondling, prolonged gazing, and touch are barometers that have been used in an effort to describe and measure attachment behavior. These activities involve both opportunity and ability on the part of the mother and infant. The infant's sensory and motor abilities evoke responses from the mother and begin the communication that is especially helpful for proper attachment to begin. Stern (1971) has observed that patterns of interaction between a mother and her child have a characteristic rhythm. Intricate interchanges take place within a few minutes. If these interactions are interrupted for any reason, or are not allowed to form, many aspects of the relationship between the two individuals are disturbed. This interdependency of rhythms seems to be at the root of mother-child attachment as well as of early communicative behaviors.

A lack of attachment during the early months can translate into later caregiving deficiencies. These deficiencies can be made worse if the child is ill for a prolonged period. A wide range of stressful factors may take place during pregnancy and the neonatal period that can profoundly influence a woman's subsequent mothering behavior and, ultimately, her child's developmental outcome. Parents lose much when their infant is born prematurely or when their child is medically fragile during the first year of life. Taylor and Hall (1979) point out that parents of premature or critically ill infants face unexpected realities. These realities include the realization that

1. A scrawny, underweight, high-risk infant, who is either seriously ill or likely to become so, replaces the expected healthy full-term infant.
2. An underreactive or underactive infant replaces the responsive and reactive infant with whom the parents had expected to interact actively.
3. Separation replaces the frequent close contact between parents and infant.
4. An incubator in a sophisticated intensive care or hospital unit replaces the expected bassinet beside the mother's bed.
5. Nurses and physicians (strangers) replace the parents as primary caregivers.
6. The mother especially has failed to produce the expected baby; hence the parent's perception of failure and its accompanying loss of self-esteem replace the expected success and increase in self-esteem.

Clinical observations reporting an increased incidence of family disintegration, child abuse, failure to thrive, abandonment, and other family problems in the high-risk population have been available for years (Rossetti, 1986). More recent observations have pointed out the importance of early maternal-infant attachment for the formation of optimal caregiving routines (Pinata, Sroufe, and Egeland, 1989; Affleck, Tennen, Rowe, Roscher, and Walker, 1989; Donovan and Leavitt, 1989; Korner et al., 1989). Clearly, there is a need to detect the patterns of attachment that may be indicative of impending deficiencies in caregiving ability.

Avant (1982) describes an assessment strategy designed to focus on maternal attachment behaviors. The assessment scale consists of a one-page observation checklist. The overall purpose of the scale is to provide a simple and systematic method of observing maternal behavior. The scale consists of a list of common attachment behaviors, compiled from several sources, that can be observed early in the child's life (during a newborn feeding period). Four sets of scores are yielded: overall attachment, affectionate behavior, proximity maintaining, and caretaking. Table 6-5 presents a modification of the score sheet used on the scale.

What this scale and others like it provide is an opportunity to observe, in a structured manner, behaviors on which normal attachment can be judged. If normal attachment patterns are detected, then the probability of normal interactional patterns developing is increased. In the absence of normal attachment, the risk of deficient interactional patterns is increased, along with the risk of later communicative pathology.

Play Behavior

The relationship between symbolic play and language has been the focus of much recent attention. A number of developmental consistencies between play and language may be observed in normally developing children. Change in play complexity is accompanied by concurrent changes in lan-

TABLE 6-5. Maternal-infant observation scale

Affectionate behavior subscale	Proximity maintaining subscale
Positions infant en face	Mother holds infant
Looking at infant	Close contact with infant
Talking (singing, cooing to infant)	Encompasses infant
ATL (accessory touch/love)	Infant on mother's knee
Kisses infant	
Smiles at infant	
Touches with fingertips only	
Touches with fingertips and palms	

Source: Adapted from P. Avant (1982). A maternal attachment assessment strategy. In S. Humenick-Smith (Ed.), *Analysis of current assessment strategies in the health care of young children and childbearing families*. Norwich, CT: Appleton-Century-Crofts.

guage function and usage. The relationship between symbolic play and language development is well established (Terrell and Schwartz, 1988).

Several models for better understanding play behavior have been suggested. One, described by Mindes (1982), is presented in Table 6-6. This model looks at three broad categories of play (social, cognitive, and miscellaneous play) with several subcategories under each main heading. Although this information is not in an assessment format, it can assist the assessor in gaining a better understanding of the nature of play and of the different functions play performs in the developing child.

The concept of measuring play behavior is a relatively new one. Several instruments are designed to describe and label play behavior. In recent years a growing body of evidence has demonstrated not only the variability of infant behavior but also the extent to which children exert control over

TABLE 6-6. Definitions of play categories

SOCIAL PLAY

Solitary play: The child plays alone with toys different from those used by other children; the child is centered on self-activity

Parallel play: The child plays independently but among other children; the child plays beside rather than with other children

Group play–associative play: The child plays with other children; all engage in similar if not identical activity

Cooperative play: The child plays in an organized group; there is a sense of belonging and an organization in which the efforts of one child are supplemented by the other children

COGNITIVE PLAY

Functional play: Simple muscular activities and repetitive muscular movements with or without objects are used in functional play; the child repeats or initiates actions

Constructive play: The child learns the use of play materials and attempts to create something with play materials

Dramatic play: The child takes on a role and pretends to be someone else using real or imagined objects

Games with rules: The child accepts and adjusts to prearranged rules

MISCELLANEOUS PLAY

Unoccupied behavior: The child is not playing in the usual sense but watches activities of momentary interest

Onlooker behavior: The child watches others play

Reading: The child is being read to by an adult caregiver.

Source: Adapted from G. Mindes (1982). Social and cognitive aspects of play in young handicapped children. *Topics of Early Childhood Special Education, 2,* 14.

their environment (Als, 1977). There have been numerous attempts to categorize the variability and sophistication of behavioral responses in infants, some of which have been previously mentioned. However, attempts to quantify play behavior are only now emerging.

Several researchers have developed scales to assess the developmental progression of play. The *Manual for Analyzing Free Play* (MAFP), proposed by McCune-Nicolich (1980), incorporates a play sequence initially suggested by Piaget (1962). The MAFP includes strategies for categorizing symbolic, relational, and manipulative play. In categorizing symbolic play a series of discrete judgments is made by the assessor concerning the child's play behavior. The instrument provides a flowchart that assists the examiner in better determining the overall level of the play behaviors observed. Table 6-7 presents an adapted version of the play levels (symbolic play) and specific play behaviors incorporated as part of the MAFP. Manipulative and relational play are coded in a similar manner.

Additional paradigms for charting the development of play from a Piagetian standpoint are provided by Smilansky (1968); Lowe (1975); Belsky and Most (1981); Rubin, Maioni, and Hornung (1976); Enslein and Fein (1981); Uzgiris and Hunt (1975); and Dunst (1980).

Westby (1980) presented information regarding the assessment of cognitive and language abilities through play. The Westby data linked play activities with concurrent language skills that should be expected at various ages. A sample of the play activities and concurrent language behaviors expected is presented in Table 6-8.

An additional description of developmental change in play behavior seen as a function of age was provided by Largo and Howard (1979), who described three different types of play behavior — with exploratory, with functional, and with spatial characteristics. Table 6-9 presents an adaptation of the Largo and Howard data.

The observation of play activity using the formats suggested above and others assists the practitioner in monitoring the way the child develops representational thought. A large body of evidence relates certain cognitive attainments to various features of language development. Although no one-to-one mapping of language onto cognition exists, it is clear that certain play behaviors reflect cognitive skills necessary as precursors to the development of spoken language. Language and play both require that a child mentally represent reality. Just as a child must realize that a doll is only a representation of a live baby or that a piece of paper can serve as a child's blanket, so must he or she understand that a word is not the object but only a representation of the object. Hence, the practitioner must be familiar with the concept of play assessment and how play affects language development.

TABLE 6-7. Categorizing symbolic play

Level	Play behaviors
Level 1: presymbolic scheme	Child picks up comb, touches it to hair, drops it
	Child picks up telephone, puts it to ear, sets it aside
	Child gives mop a swish on floor
	Child hammers
	Child rolls truck on floor
Level 2: autosymbolic scheme	Child simulates drinking form a toy baby bottle
	Child eats from an empty spoon
	Child closes eyes and pretends to sleep
Level 3: single-scheme symbolic games	Child feeds mother or doll
	Child grooms mother or doll
	Child pretends to read a book
	Child pretends to mop floor
Level 4-1: single-scheme combinations	Child combs own, then mother's, hair
	Child drinks from bottle, then feeds doll from bottle
	Child cleans several objects with sponge
Level 4-2: multischeme combinations	Child holds telephone to ear, dials, then talks
	Child kisses doll, puts it to bed, puts spoon to its mouth
	Child stirs in the pot, feeds doll, pours food into dish
Levels 5-1 and 5-2: planned symbolic sets and combinations	Child picks up bottle, says "baby," then feeds the doll and covers it with cloth
	Child finds iron, sets it down, searches for cloth, then irons (5-1)
	Child puts play foods in pot, stirs, says "mommy" or "soup," then feeds mother (5-2)
	Child picks up play screwdriver, says "toothbrush," and makes the motion of toothbrush

Source: Adapted from L. McCune-Nicolich (1980). *A manual for analyzing free play* (Exp. Ed.). New Brunswick, NJ: Rutgers University.

TABLE 6-8. Symbolic play scale checklist

Play activity	Language
STAGE I: 9-12 MONTHS	
Awareness that objects exist when not seen	No true language; may have words associated with some actions
Does not mouth or bang all toys	Exhibits some command and request behaviors
STAGE II: 13-17 MONTHS	
Purposeful exploration of toys; discovers operation of toys through trial and error	Single words used (context dependent)
Hands toy to adult if unable to operate on own	Communicative functions include request, command, response, greeting, protesting
STAGE III: 17-19 MONTHS	
Child pretends to go to sleep or drink from cup	Beginning of true verbal communication
STAGE IV: 19-22 MONTHS	
Symbolic play extends beyond the child's self	Beginning of word combinations with following semantic relations
Child plays with dolls, combines two toys in play, performs pretend activities	
STAGE V: 24 MONTHS	
Represents daily experiences, plays house, uses objects in a realistic manner	Uses increased phrases and short sentences
	Following morphologic markers appear: "ing" endings, plurals, possessives
STAGE VI: 30 MONTHS	
Represents events less frequently experienced	Responds to WH questions: what, who, whose, where
	Asks WH questions
STAGE VII: 36 MONTHS	
Obvious sequence to play activities	Uses past tense
Associative play	Uses future aspects (particularly "gonna") such as "I'm gonna wash dishes."
Reenactment of events with varying outcomes	

Source: Adapted from C. Westby (1980). Assessment of cognitive and language abilities through play. *Language Speech and Hearing Services in the Schools, 3,* 154.

TABLE 6-9. Developmental progression in play behavior

Behavior category	Age (mo)
PLAY BEHAVIOR WITH EXPLORATORY CHARACTERISTICS	
Mouthing: object is brought to the mouth and explored with the lips and tongue	9-15
Manipulatory play: object is visually examined, fingered, and turned	1-18
PLAY BEHAVIOR WITH FUNCTIONAL CHARACTERISTICS	
Functional play: object is used in an appropriate manner; play is restricted to the child's own body	9-18
Representational play I: object is used in a functionally appropriate way, but with play directed toward another person	12-30
Representational play II: doll is manipulated by child; child uses objects in a functionally appropriate manner	21-30
Sequential play: sequence of play behavior occurs inside a common framework	21-30
Symbolic play: object is symbolically substituted for an absent one	30+
PLAY BEHAVIOR WITH SPATIAL CHARACTERISTICS	
Relational play: objects are brought in touch with each other in a nonfunctional way	9-15
Container play: one object is put into another in a nonfunctional manner	9-15
Stacking: objects are placed one on another	18-21
Grouping: same type of objects are clustered	15-24
Spatial arrangement: objects are placed on chairs, tables, dishes	18-30

Source: Adapted from H. Largo and J. Howard (1979). Developmental progression in play behavior of children between nine and thirty months: Spontaneous play and imitation. *Developmental Medicine and Child Neurology, 21, 299.*

Pragmatics

When a speaker uses language to affect others or to relay information, the speaker uses pragmatics. *Pragmatics* can be defined as a set of sociolinguistic rules related to language use within the communicative context. That is, pragmatics is concerned with the way language is used to communicate rather than the way language is structured (Owens, 1988).

In general, children learn language within the conversational context. During the preschool years the child acquires many conversational skills. Much of the child's language during these years concerns the here and now, and much regarding the accepted routines of conversation has yet to be learned. In general, the 2-year-old child is able to respond to a conversational partner and to engage in short dialogues of a few turns on a given topic. The child can also introduce a change in the topic of discussion. By age 3 years, he or she can engage in longer conversations beyond a few turns. As the 3-year-old child becomes more aware of the social aspects of discourse, he or she better acknowledges the partner's turn. By kindergarten the child has learned the basic rules for the social usage of language. However, pragmatic learning continues for some time.

The learning of pragmatic rules is set in motion initially by the nature of the interactions that take place between mother (primary caregiver) and infant. In reviewing the characteristics of mother-infant talk it becomes readily apparent that the nature of mother-infant talk sets in motion a variety of learning processes, one of which is pragmatics. Olswang, Stoel-Gammons, Coggins, and Carpenter (1987) present eight characteristics of mother-infant talk (Table 6-10). A review of these characteristics readily reveals how conducive they are to the development of pragmatic functions.

In any area of development that is tied to maturational processes, measurement is possible. Thus, the monitoring of pragmatic development in infants and toddlers is possible. Antoniadis, Didow, Lockhart, and Moroge (1984) present information regarding screening for early cognitive and communicative behaviors. In the data from Antoniadis's group, a scale for screening social communication–pragmatics is provided. No normative data is used; however, the scale is quite helpful as the practitioner attempts to structure observations of social-pragmatic use of language by the infant or toddler. Table 6-11 presents a sample of the behaviors included in the scale.

In an additional discussion of the communicative skills of infants and toddlers, Chapman (1981) assigned communicative performance to a series of

TABLE 6-10. Characteristics of mother-infant talk

1. Short utterance length and simple syntax
2. Object-centered small core vocabulary
3. Topics limited to here and now
4. Heightened use of facial expression and gestures
5. Frequent questioning and greeting
6. Infant behaviors are treated as meaningful: mother awaits infant's turn and responds even to nonturns
7. Frequent (paralinguistic) modifications of pitch and loudness
8. Frequent verbal rituals

Source: Adapted from L. Olswang, C. Stoel-Gammons, T. Coggins, and R. Carpenter (1987). *Assessing linguistic behaviors.* Seattle: University of Washington Press.

**TABLE 6-11. Social communication —
Pragmatics screening items**

Age (mo)	Behaviors
0-9	Intracommunicative behaviors such as cry, touch, smile, vocal, grasp, suck, laugh
0-9	Reciprocal gesture
9-18	Demonstrates communicative intent by Pointing to objects Showing objects Giving objects
9-18	Regulates behavior of self and others
9-18	Protests (voice or gesture)
9-18	Verbal turn-taking
18-24	Engages in adultlike dialogue
18-24	Uses language to pretend
18-24	Uses language to control and interact with others

Source: Adapted from A. Antoniadis, S. Didow, S. Lockhart, and P. Moroge (1984). Screening for early cognitive and communicative behaviors. *Communique, 9,* 14.

phases. Chapman demonstrated that children use gestural means of communication at 12 to 18 months of age; gestures plus wordlike vocalizations at 12 to 18 months; conventional words or word combinations to express a range of intentions at 18 to 24 months; requests for objects, or action, rejections, or protest at 18 to 24 months; and a variety of newly developed intentions (discourse functions) at 18 to 24 months. These behaviors indicate that the child has now incorporated some of the basic rules of conversation into a communicative repertoire, such as the rule indicating the obligation to respond to speech in an appropriate manner.

Kiernan (1986) lists several behaviors that relate to the child's ability to display social behaviors without a direct communicative intent. These reflect the child's growing awareness of the manner in which a variety of behaviors fit within the social context in which the child resides. A sampling of these behaviors is contained in Figure 6-2.

Weatherby and Prizant (1988) described a recently designed instrument intended to detect early communication problems in infants and toddlers. The *Communication and Symbolic Behavior Scales* (CSBS) is an assessment tool designed to examine the communication, social, affective, and symbolic abilities of children functioning between a 9-month-old and a 2-year-old communication age (Weatherby and Prizant, 1989). The authors indicate that the CSBS has a twofold purpose. First, it is used for early identification of children who have or are at risk for developing communication

BEHAVIOR	USUALLY	RARELY	NEVER
1. Child watches other people with interest.	☐	☐	☐
2. Child responds differently to familiar people and to strangers (e.g., by smiling, moving closer, or showing excitement to familiar people).	☐	☐	☐
3. Child sits beside, snuggles up to, or touches a familiar person.	☐	☐	☐
4. Child initiates eye contact with another person when that person is near.	☐	☐	☐
5. Child hovers by another person for attention (but does not touch or try to make contact or make attention-getting sounds).	☐	☐	☐

Figure 6-2. Social interaction without communication. (Adapted from L. Kiernan [1986]. Preverbal communication schedule. Unpublished manuscript.)

impairment. Second, it is designed to establish a profile of communication and symbolic and effective communication to assist in future assessment and plan intervention. The authors indicate that the CSBS will be published in experimental form in 1989 and field tested across the United States. It is expected that the CSBS in final form will be available for general use in 1990 or 1991. It is precisely such efforts, put forth by innovative investigators such as Weatherby and Prizant, that will serve to enhance further the assessor's ability to detect and monitor communicative delay and performance in infants and toddlers.

Assessment of Gestures

The use of gestures as a precursor to verbal communication makes it possible for the practitioner to structure observations to monitor gestural development and usage. Several current assessment instruments have sections that require the assessor to note the presence or absence of various age-related gestures. Although normative data, in the context of test administration, are limited regarding gestural usage, there are ample data describing the presence of gestures at various ages.

One paradigm that is helpful in monitoring gesture development and change is provided by Olswang, Stoel-Gammons, Coggins, and Carpenter

(1987). A language and gesture inventory is provided as part of the *Assessing Prelinguistic and Early Linguistic Behaviors in Young Children* test battery. Gesture behaviors are listed in six distinct categories, and the assessor simply indicates whether a particular behavior is present. The six categories are (1) social regulation and social games, (2) greetings, signs of affection, and bedtime, (3) eating and drinking, (4) dressing, grooming, and washing, (5) adult activities, and (6) toys and games. This instrument represents the first comprehensive attempt to structure gestural assessment as part of a complete battery designed to assess prelinguistic and early linguistic skills. A sample of the specific behaviors included in the gesture inventory is provided in Table 6-12.

An additional format described for measuring gestural communication is provided by Kiernan (1986) as part of a comprehensive intrument designed to measure preverbal communication skills. The instrument, known as the *Preverbal Communication Schedule* (PVC), is described by the author as being applicable for use with infants or with those children who display little speech or language behavior. Although the norms provided with the PVC were obtained on populations of mentally handicapped persons, the subscales are useful in monitoring gestural usage and development. Figure 6-3 presents an adapted form of the gestural subscale of the PVC.

Coplan (1987) incorporates gestural assessment into the *Early Language Milestone Scale* (ELM). The ELM was created to provide interested professionals with a rapid and reliable way to assess language development in children 0 to 3 years of age. Part of the developmental profile obtained on children through administration of the ELM relates to the use of gestures. The data may be obtained from parental report. Coplan suggests that the easiest way to gain needed information is to ask the parents, "Does your baby ever play peek-a-boo or pat-a-cake or wave bye-bye?" If parents respond in the affirmative, then the parents are asked whether the child demonstrates these behaviors spontaneously or imitatively.

Two instruments that are designed specifically to assess early language skills and that incorporate gestural items are the *Oliver* (MacDonald, 1979) and the *Environmental Prelanguage Battery* (Horstmeier and MacDonald, 1978). Several test items relating to gesture are built into these instruments and used when computing an overall score for language ability and development. The *Early Intervention Developmental Profile* (EIDP) is another instrument that incorporates gestural items as part of an overall assessment of children 0 to 36 months of age (Rogers, 1987). The EIDP is designed to gather data on children's cognitive, motor, social, self-care, and language skills. It is receiving widespread usage because of its comprehensive nature, which crosses several developmental domains.

Gesture assessment permits the assessor to structure observations of gesture more completely during infant-toddler assessments. The absence of ges-

TABLE 6-12. Gesture inventory behaviors

SOCIAL REGULATION AND SOCIAL GAMES

"Up" (arms reaching upward in request to be picked up)

Showing (extends arm toward other with object in hand)

Peek-a-boo (covers and uncovers face)

Nods head yes

"All gone" (shrugs and puts out hands in gesture of surprise)

GREETINGS, SIGNS OF AFFECTION, BEDTIME

Waves hi/bye

Hugs (dolls, people, or animals)

Puts to bed (puts dolls, people, or animals in bed)

Rocks (dolls, people, or animals)

EATING AND DRINKING

Drinking (brings container to mouth)

Feeding others (puts utensil to mouth of others/doll)

Wipes (wipes hands or face with napkin or bib)

Pouring (makes gesture of pouring from a container)

DRESSING, GROOMING, AND WASHING

Combs or brushes hair

Brushes teeth

Hat (puts on or tries to put on)

Diapering (takes off/puts on diapers, powders bottom)

ADULT ACTIVITIES

Telephone (puts receiver to ear)

Pushes stroller or shopping cart

Musical instrument (tries to play an instrument)

Writing or typing

TOYS AND GAMES

Ball (throws or kicks ball)

Car/truck (rolls or pushes toy vehicles)

Gun/pistol (makes a shooting gesture)

Airplane (makes a gesture of flying an airplane or helicopter in the air)

Source: Adapted from L. Olswang, C. Stoel–Gammon, T. Coggins, and R. Carpenter (1987). *Assessing linguistic behaviors.* Seattle: University of Washington Press.

BEHAVIOR	USUALLY	RARELY	NEVER
Reaches out to be lifted	☐	☐	☐
Shakes head yes or no	☐	☐	☐
Waves good-bye without prompting	☐	☐	☐
Gestures to indicate needs (pretends to drink)	☐	☐	☐
Gestures regarding toileting needs	☐	☐	☐

Figure 6-3. Communication through gestures. (Adapted from L. Kiernan [1986]. Preverbal communication schedule. Unpublished manuscript.)

ture behaviors may indicate impending language deficits. These may become more obvious and pronounced at a later date, when more traditional language milestones are expected. Although additional research on gesture is needed, enough information exists to permit the assessor to use gesture as an important part of a complete assessment of the language domain.

The clinician working with infants and toddlers is wise to incorporate the observation of some of the above-mentioned behaviors into a comprehensive assessment of the child's overall communicative ability. Although overlap exists between the behaviors outlined in the previous section and those listed under other communicative functions, the overlap noted is not necessarily negative. Rather, it ensures that the assessor is gaining a more complete picture of all communicative behaviors as an attempt is made to provide data on general communicative skills and abilities.

Language Comprehension and Expression

Delayed development of speech and language are the most common symptoms of developmental disability in childhood, affecting somewhere between 5 and 10 percent of all children and 69 percent of all 3- to 5-year-old children receiving early intervention services. In populations of children at known risk for developmental deficit, the percentage of children who display some form of communicative deficit is substantially higher. Coplan (1985) reinforces this view by stating that in the course of the normal day a pediatrician will see at least one or two children with communicative deficits. Given the prevalence of communicative deficits in children 0 to 3 years of age, it is imperative that the practitioner become familiar with procedures for assessing speech and language development.

The areas under discussion thus far have concentrated on various aspects of communicative performance that are more recent in assessment. These areas are receiving considerable attention from both the clinical and theoretical standpoint. This attention is created in large measure by the resurgence of interest in infant development as well as by the mandate (see Chap. 1) to provide early intervention services to younger and younger children. A more traditional view of speech and language assessment has viewed the main aspects of language as language comprehension and expression skills. Hence, the information to follow will discuss the assessment of language comprehension and expression in children.

Language comprehension. There is a strong link between cognition, comprehension, and production in child language. Children learn language by first determining, independent of language, the meaning a speaker intends to convey to them and by then working out the relationship between the meaning and the language (Macnamara, 1972). Thus, as children pass through various stages of growth in language comprehension, they should display behaviors reflecting this process. These behaviors constitute the basis for measuring language comprehension.

When evaluating very young children with delayed language, the assessor may not be able to rely totally on parental impressions about the child's comprehension skills. Children with delayed language use strategies that make them appear to understand language, when in fact their comprehension is based on attention paid to nonlinguistic behaviors and cues such as gaze, gestures, or event probabilities (Paul and Fischer, 1986; Tager-Flusberg, 1981).

There are very few standardized tests of language comprehension for children under 3 years of age. Of those available, the majority assess single-word vocabulary. Examples of instruments of this nature include the *Peabody Picture Vocabulary Test* (Dunn and Dunn, 1981), the *Receptive One Word Picture Vocabulary Test* (Gardner, 1979), and the *Vocabulary Comprehension Scale* (Bangs, 1975). Other more general instruments, such as the *Receptive-Expressive Emergent Language Scale* (Bzoch and League, 1971) and the *Sequenced Inventory of Communicative Development* (Hedrick, Prather, and Tobin, 1975), look at a range of responses to verbal and nonverbal auditory stimuli. Although these general measures can be quite useful for assessing listening skills, more specific information about the way children process word combinations and sentences is needed (Paul and Fischer, 1985).

Any assessment of language comprehension must be concerned with the child's ability to understand language apart from the types of nonlinguistic cues mentioned previously. The presence of this ability, specifically behaviors that demonstrate comprehension apart from cues, must be identified observationally. This can become difficult since the vocabulary items included on standard tests may not be part of the child's comprehension repertoire. For example, the child may have appropriate comprehension skills. However, the items that the child is readily able to comprehend may be items peculiar to the child's individual environment and not be part of a standard test battery of items. Paul and Fischer (1985) suggest that the practitioner should briefly interview parents by telephone regarding the child's comprehension skills. Parents can then be asked to bring to the evaluation several items whose name the child might know. This is a very helpful suggestion and one to which the experienced assessor will readily attest.

An additional caution should be expressed at this point. The assessor is interested in determining overall comprehension status. As such, all behaviors indicating the child's ability to comprehend meaning (whether supported by the usual temporal, contextual, and gestural cues), as well as comprehension expressed through understanding of vocabulary items, are of interest to the examiner. As the examiner is able to control the cues available to the child, the specific type of comprehension ability demonstrated by the child can be better monitored.

The task for the assessor, regardless of the particular assessment instrument used, if any, is to determine the child's language comprehension ability. The types of cues provided the child during the assessment must be controlled carefully by the examiner. Thus the assessor must be alert to procedures that are cue free. Behaviors that the practitioner must learn to avoid include looking at the object being named, pointing toward the desired object, or identifying an object the child is already holding.

Several researchers have developed checklists of words likely to be comprehended by children during the second year. These checklists have been used as corroborative data for observational studies and have proved useful as a basis for measures of individual differences in language development (Bates, Bretherton, and Snyder, 1987). Although some reservations have been expressed regarding the use of vocabulary checklists as a valid index of child language, there is reasonable support for the claim that vocabulary checklists are valid instruments for assessing aspects of child language (Reznick and Goldsmith, 1988). In support of the supposition that vocabulary checklists can be used as a valid index of language comprehension, a variety of researchers have undertaken investigations designed to do so. Basically, these researchers have found that child performance on vocabulary checklist tasks is significantly correlated with scores on the *Bayley Scale of Infant Development* and the *Peabody Picture Vocabulary Test* at 13 and 24 months of age (Olson, Bates, and Bayles, 1982). Reznick (1982) used vocabulary checklists for 8-, 14-, and 20-month-old children and found a reasonable pattern of similarity between parents' assessment of child language and the child's behavior in a word-comprehension procedure administered in a laboratory setting. Finally, Dale, Bates, Reznick, and Morisset (1987) gathered data on

five groups of 20-month-old children. Results report strong validity correlations with the Bayley scales and particularly with a language subscale
derived from the Bayley scales.

What these results indicate is that the use of comprehension tasks that
include items appropriate for the child's age and environment that are free
from nonlinguistic cues during administration can be a valuable means of
assessing overall language comprehension for children below 3 years
of age.

Rowan and Johnson (1988) presented information on a speech and language screening instrument in use at the University of Illinois that presents
data regarding comprehension behaviors for children birth through 12
months of age. The instrument lists specific behaviors and how these behaviors were observed. The range of possible observational categories
include parental report, observations made by the examiner, and observations made during direct testing. Figure 6-4 presents a sampling of comprehension items by age.

To assess language comprehension skills accurately, the practitioner
must be familiar with the normal progression of comprehension skills for
children in the birth to 3-year age group. If the assessor uses a formal
assessment instrument, the task is somewhat simplified. If the assessor uses
informal methodology, care must be taken to follow the normal progression of comprehension skills. In essence, whether a formal instrument or
informal procedures are used, a basal of comprehension ability must be established. Once a basal of skills is determined, more difficult comprehension tasks, reflecting greater comprehension ability, are examined. The
procedure continues until a ceiling of comprehension ability is determined.

One procedure that allows for the assessment of comprehension skills is
suggested by Paul and Fischer (1985). In this procedure the child is observed in an attempt to determine comprehension ability of single words
without the support of nonlinguistic cues, as previously discussed. The
child may simply be asked to respond to the question, "Where is X?" If the
objects are familiar to the child, some degree of comprehension skill
should easily be established. Once several noun items are identified in this
manner, the practitioner may then move on to verbs using basically the
same format. Words for action — those that the parents have indicated
that the child is likely to know — can be used. The procedure is simple in
that the child is given a familiar object and asked to, "Hit it, pat it, kiss it,
throw it," and so on. As Chapman (1981) has suggested, comprehension
of single words without the support of nonlinguistic cues indicates performance expected in the 12- to 18-month range. If the child is unable to
demonstrate comprehension using these formats, the clinician may wish
to support the requests made to the child with gestural (nonlinguistic)
cues. Performance in this manner suggests comprehension ability in the 8-
to 12-month range.

AGE (MO)	COMPREHENSION ITEM
0–3	
_____	Alerting response to sound
_____	Activity diminishes or ceases when approached by sound
_____	Quieted by a familiar voice
_____	Smiles at mother's voice
_____	Often watches speaker's mouth
3–6	
_____	Shows fear of angry voice
_____	Anticipates feeding at sight of food
_____	Recognizes and responds to name
_____	Appears to recognize words like "up," "bye-bye"
_____	Responds to pleasant speech by smiling
6–9	
_____	Moves toward or searches toward family member when named
_____	Begins to show recognition of "no"
_____	Begins to anticipate visual games
_____	Shows stranger anxiety
_____	Relates sound to an object
9–12	
_____	Action response to verbal request
_____	Shakes head yes or no
_____	Understands "hot" and "so big"
_____	Understands some action words
_____	Frowns when scolded
_____	May follow simple commands when given by gesture

Figure 6-4. Speech and language screening comprehension items. The items are observed in any of the following ways: PR = parental report; O = direct observation; DT = direct testing. (Adapted from L. Rowan and C. Johnson [1988]. Screening and assessment. Paper presented at the June 1988 infant and toddler communication assessment and intervention workshop, Minneapolis, MN.)

If basic comprehension is established at this level (12 to 18 months), more difficult comprehension tasks are then attempted. At this point the practitioner moves on to assess comprehension at the 18- to 24-month level. The assessment of understanding using two-word instructions is introduced at this point. The items used in previous levels of testing should be used as two-word units are assessed. Hence, the nouns previously identified by the child should be used in conjunction with the verbs previously identified. The two-word utterances used during this section of testing should be attempted several times, thus maximizing the child's opportunity to demonstrate appropriate understanding. Both familiar and unfamiliar combinations of nouns and verbs can be used at this stage of assessment. Novel combinations of action-object words can be used. It can be assumed that if the child demonstrates appropriate performance to an utterance such as "Kiss the car," appropriate comprehension is present.

Beyond the 24-month level a greater number of traditional assessment instruments exist. Appendix B describes a variety of instruments that will assist in determining comprehension ability at this stage of development. Instruments such as the *Peabody Picture Vocabulary Test* (Dunn and Dunn, 1981) the *Test of Auditory Comprehension of Language* (Carrow, 1973), the *Environmental Language Battery* (Horstmeier and MacDonald, 1978), the *Receptive-Expressive Emergent Language Scale* (Bzoch and League, 1971), or the *Miller-Yoder Test of Grammatical Comprehension* (Miller and Yoder, 1982) are good examples.

Table 6-13 presents a sequence of comprehension ability. This information was initially presented by Chapman (1981). The information presented in this table may be used by the assessor as an informal guide in structuring comprehension tasks until the child reaches the age at which more formal assessment instruments might be used as part of the assessment battery.

Three additional assessment instruments, designed for use with infants and toddlers, should be mentioned at this point. These are the *Early Language Milestone Scale* (Coplan, Gleason, Ryan, Burke, and Williams, 1982), the *Assessing Linguistic Behaviors Scale* (Olswang, Stoel-Gammon, Coggins, and Carpenter, 1987), and the *Early Language Inventory* (Bates et al., 1986). Each of these instruments uses a combination of parent reporting and direct observation to determine language comprehension ability of children under 3 years of age (see Appendix B).

Assessing language comprehension for children under 3 years of age certainly taxes the clinical judgment of even the most experienced examiner. What emerges is a paradigm that uses a combination of procedures, including the administration of parent questionnaires, direct observation of behaviors thorugh the use of informal assessment procedures, and the administration of established language comprehension evaluation instruments. It is imperative that the practitioner become an astute observer of spontaneous behaviors. It is precisely these observations that may, in part,

TABLE 6-13. Comprehension ability by age

Age (mo)	Comprehension ability	Comprehension strategy
8–12	Understands a few single words in routine context	1. Looks at objects mother looks at 2. Acts on objects noticed 3. Imitates ongoing action
12–18	Understands single words outside of routine; some contextual cues needed	1. Attends to object mentioned 2. Performs usual activities with familiar objects
18–24	Understands words for absent objects; some two-word combinations understood	1. Locates objects mentioned 2. Follows simple commands
24–36	Comprehension of three word sentences; needs context of past experience to determine meaning	1. Supplies missing information

Source: Adapted from R. Chapman (1981). Exploring children's communicative intents. In J. Miller (Ed.), *Assessing language production in children: Experimental procedures.* Baltimore: University Park Press.

provide a foundation for determining the adequacy of the child's language comprehension. Previous chapters encouraged the practitioner to have a proper understanding of the results obtained during a single assessment. These points must be paramount in the assessor's mind as language comprehension is evaluated.

Language expression. When attempting to assess language expression, the first activity undertaken should be to obtain a description of past and current behaviors. This is best obtained from the parents. It should be communicated to them how important information of this nature is, in particular if the child is at an age when traditional measures of language expression are difficult. The parents can fill out a questionnaire on the child's language usage. Several examples were given in previous sections (see Appendix A). Figure 6-5 presents a questionnaire oriented toward language-speech expression. Some of the expression items contained in Fig. 6-5 represent speech-oriented behaviors (S), while others represent communication-oriented behaviors (C).

A second methodology is to conduct a careful, communicatively oriented parent interview. A third strategy that the examiner may wish to employ is to observe the child and parents interacting in the clinic or home setting.

Age (mo)	Expression item
0–3	
_____	Reflexive cry
_____	Soft, throaty noises
_____	Begins differentiated cry
_____	Vocal sounds of pleasure
_____	Begins sustained laughter
_____	Vocalizes two or more different syllables
3–6	
_____	Talks back in face-to-face interaction (S)
_____	Produces more vowels than consonants (S)
_____	Vocalizes to objects that move (S)
_____	Protests when objects are removed (S)
_____	Initiates simple person-oriented acts (C)
6–9	
_____	Initiates "conversations" with toys (C)
_____	Babbles using many different phonemes (S)
_____	Inconsistently imitates noises of others (S)
_____	Shakes head "no" (C)
_____	Expresses desire by hand gesture (C)
9–12	
_____	Echoes speech and imitates sound (C)
_____	Copies melody pattern of familiar phrases (S)
_____	Tugs on mother for attention (C)
_____	Initiates speech games (S)
_____	Uses one to three words (C)

Figure 6-5. Speech and language screening expression items. The items are observed in any of the following ways: PR = parental report; O = direct observation; DT = direct testing. (Adapted from L. Rowan and C. Johnson [1988]. Screening and assessment. Paper presented at the June 1988 infant and toddler communication assessment and intervention workshop, Minneapolis, MN.)

Special attention can be paid to the expressive language the child displays. A combination of all three of these methods — child questionnaire, an interview, and direct observation of parent-child interaction — provides the most complete and useful body of information about the child's past and present language expression. These activities are not intended to supplant the need to use formal assessment instruments. However, the assessor must be aware that instruments designed to measure language expression in children under 3 years of age are in an emerging state. At no time should parent information, or behavior observed by the assessor, be overlooked or undervalued in the presence of contradictory test results.

In many instances the major source of information about a child's language expression ability will be through direct observations of the child. These observations may be structured or unstructured. Regardless, they are based in part on what is known about the normal progression of language expression seen in normally developing children. It is crucial that the samples of behavior on which decisions are made be as representative as possible. The issue of representativeness must be a major consideration in choosing assessment techniques and instruments. Procedures for structuring observations of child language performance can be divided into two main categories: structured and unstructured. Each will be discussed in the information to follow.

Structured (standard) tests of language expression. Standardized tests provide a specific set of instructions and stimuli to elicit behaviors and a specific set of standards for scoring and interpreting elicited behaviors (Bernstine and Tiegerman, 1985, p. 122). Usually the standards for interpretation are norms based on a sample population's performance on the test stimuli. A child's performance on a test can be compared with the norms obtained from the standardized sample in one of two ways, yielding an age-equivalent score or a score of relative standing. The focus in most standardized tests is on a child's total or overall score.

Standardized tests of this nature can be valuable during an initial assessment to determine whether the child's performance is within developmental expectations. However, the outcome of this type of measure rarely provides the kind of comprehensive, in-depth information required for planning an intervention program. That is not to say that these results do not assist the practitioner in addressing intervention issues. However, prescriptive guidance regarding specific intervention activities is usually not provided. Chapter 5 presented more detailed information on the various types of tests available to the assessor. Appendix B lists a variety of structured assessment instruments covering language and additional developmental domains.

Nonstandard expressive language assessment procedures. Nonstandard procedures are not synonymous with informal or unstructured observations.

They differ from standard procedures or tests in that they do not have a
well-established set of stimuli or instructions that must be adhered to, nor
do they have well-established standards or norms for interpretation. They
do have sufficient face validity to be used in assessing various aspects of language, and they include a mix of structured tasks and unstructured observations. One of the primary assets of nonstandard procedures is that they are
flexible and can be adapted to fit the needs and characteristics of the child
being evaluated. Because the assessor is not locked into a particular stimu-
lus or method for eliciting information, a child's knowledge and abilities
can be explored by varying content, form, and presentation of the stimuli.
Nonstandard procedures include collection and analysis of spontaneous
language samples and techniques for eliciting production of particular
aspects of language usage.

A good example of a nonstandard assessment instrument is the *Infant
Scale of Communicative Intent* (1982) (ISCI). The ISCI is designed as a
nonstandardized, descriptive measure developed to meet the needs of a
population of infants with developmental problems. Items on the scale are
administered by observation, direct testing, or parental reporting and are
scored on a pass-fail basis. This scale has value in that it allows for the
collection of data on the child's expressive ability in several ways. The scale
has a comprehension and an expression section. Table 6-14 represents an
adapted form of the language portion of the scale.

Two additional nonstandard measures of language expression are reported by Reznick and Goldsmith (1988) and by Dale, Bates, Reznick, and
Morriset (1988). These involve a multiple-form word production checklist
for assessing early language and a parent reporting instrument of child language at 20 months of age, respectively. The Reznick and Goldsmith study
suggests that obtaining a sample vocabulary (based on an adaptation of the
Communicative Development Inventory) is well correlated with other
normed measures of language expression ability. Five lists of vocabulary
items were used. These lists were divided into 19 semantic categories: activities, animals, body parts, clothing, food and drinks, furniture and rooms,
household, outside, people, places to go, prepositions, pronouns, qualities,
quantifiers, questions, time, toys, vehicles, and verbs (auxilliary).

The language production checklists were mailed to parents who had
agreed to participate in the study. The age range of the children was 11 to
24 months. Results indicated that parental responses to the lists reflected
age-related changes in production vocabulary. Furthermore, a significant correlation was observed between vocabulary performance on this abbreviated
task and language expression instruments of greater length and complexity.
The authors conclude by stating that when an assessor needs a single estimate of a child's production vocabulary when production vocabulary must
be monitored longitudinally, or when time or parental cooperation are concerns, the procedures used in the investigation are an acceptable option.

TABLE 6-14. Infant scale of communicative intent

Age (mo)	Language expression items	Age (mo)	Language expression items
0-1	Undifferentiated cry for needs Vegetative vocalizations Nasalized vowels Fake cry — bid for attention	9-10	Intentional communication Gestures with vocalization Sounds used to call others
1-2	Beginning of differentiated cry Gurgles in response to stimulation Produces short vowel sounds Cries for social stimulation	10-11	Vocabulary of two words Uses objects as tools Laughs at own sounds Attempts to label objects
2-3	Definite cooing Glottal-velar consonants Turn-taking Alert to people	11-12	May recognize words as symbols Uses "ma-ma" with meaning Imitates new sounds Imitates some tones sung by adult
3-4	Initiates babbling Chuckles — short of vocalized laugh Whines for manipulation Vocalizes feelings of pleasure	12-13	Uses four meaningful words Immature jargon used Imitates animal sounds Wakes with a "call" rather than a cry
4-5	Vocalizes laughter Vocalizes eagerness Cries if play disrupted Actively engages adult in interaction	13-14	Six-word vocabulary Points to desired object Tries to sing Imitates other children
5-6	Vocalizes "ah-goo" Imitates own noises Vocalizes to interrupt others	14-15	Up to eight-word vocabulary Initiates give and take with adults Early use of modifier
6-7	Imitates familiar sounds Expresses anger by sounds Initiates social contact Tries to imitate facial expression	15-16	Starts using double syllable words May label pictures Pulls at wet pants or diaper Pulls adult hand to show something
7-8	Reduplicated babbling Imitates sound sequence Imitates gestures Vocalizes satisfaction	16-17	Mature jargoning Differentiated object names Gradual increase in vocabulary May ask "What's that?"
8-9	Shakes head "no-no" Combines two or more consonants Shouts for attention	17-18	Up to 20-word vocabulary Ask for "more" Successive single word utterances

Source: Adapted from Update Pediatrics (1982). *An assessment tool: The infant scale of communicative intent, 7,* 1.

Dale and Bates (1987) report on the validity of a parent reporting instrument relative to assessing child language in a population of 20-month-old children. The authors feel that parent reporting is valuable as a basis for rapid overall evaluation of child language, either for screening or educational purposes. Two main conclusions may be drawn from the results of the Dale and Bates study. First, parent report measures of child language performance at 20 months of age are useful. Significant correlations between parent report data and a subscale of language performance derived from the mental scale of the *Bayley Scales of Infant Development* and the *Peabody Picture Vocabulary Test* were present. A second outcome of the Dale and Bates study was that a low relationship between socioeconomic status and vocabulary was observed. This finding suggests that the procedures used were useful across a wide range of social class. Literacy is not required of the parent, since the vocabulary list can be read to the parents. The authors conclude by stating that the checklist used can serve as a valuable component of procedures designed to detect delayed language performance in children under 3 years of age.

Language sampling. A final method that has received widespread use as a means of assessing language expression ability is language sampling. Although the child's age must be kept in mind when considering language sampling, certainly this procedure may be used any time after the child begins to demonstrate expressive ability. The first step in analyzing language production is to obtain samples of the child's productive language. Some have argued that when collected appropriately, the language sample may constitute the most accurate picture of the child's production ability (Stickler, 1987). Gallagher (1983) indicates that language sampling is the centerpiece of child language assessment.

One concept that must be kept in mind regarding language sampling relates to the representativeness of the sample obtained. A representative sample has been defined as one that is reliable and valid (Miller, 1981), one that reflects the child's optimal performance (McLean and Snyder-McLean, 1978), one that portrays the child's usual performance (Gallagher, 1983), and one that includes the child's usual productive language ability, including performance that may be somewhat below or above usual abilities (Stickler, 1987). Regardless of definition, a sample of the child's productive language must be obtained for a sufficient language analysis to be completed.

Stickler (1987) suggests that several points must be kept in mind as language samples are obtained. These relate to the nature of the interaction, the setting in which the interaction takes place, the materials used to elicit the sample, the size of the sample obtained, and the method of recording the sample. Table 6-15 presents several guidelines suggested by Stickler in

TABLE 6-15. Interaction guidelines in obtaining language samples

1. Begin with parallel play and parallel talk.
2. Move into interactive conversation.
3. Continue on the topic expressed by the child.
4. Use restricted use of questions (one question for every four speaking turns).
5. Provide options to the child that are expressed as alternative questions: "Should we play gas station or have a picnic?"
6. Use utterances that are for the most part slightly longer than the child's.
7. Learn to be comfortable with pauses in the conversation.
8. Have a variety of materials available.
9. Do not be afraid to be silly and to have fun.

Source: Adapted from K. Stickler (1987). *Guide to analysis of language transcripts.* Eau Claire, WI: Thinking Publications.

interacting with children when obtaining a language sample. Formats for analyzing expressive language samples obtained have been suggested by Miller (1981), Stickler (1987), Lee (1974), and Wig and Seml (1984).

Summary of Language Assessment for Infants and Toddlers

A variety of issues have been raised concerning assessment of the language ability of infants and toddlers. These issues include aspects of performance that are linked to later language ability as shown in recent research. Although some of these areas of assessment, such as interaction, play, gestures, and attachment, are not traditionally part of a comprehensive language assessment, deficiencies in these areas have an established link to later language deficits.

It is imperative that the assessor become familiar with procedures that are applicable and necessary to provide comprehensive language assessment for the children served. Just as new strategies have emerged over the past five years to assist in monitoring language development and detect language delay, a steady stream of innovative techniques and strategies will continue to emerge. These activities reflect the degree to which clinicians have become aware of the sensitivity of language performance as an indicator of impending developmental pathology. A comprehensive developmental evaluation of children under 3 years of age cannot be accomplished apart from assessing the language domain and paying particular attention to the aspects of language performance mentioned in the preceding section.

MOTOR DOMAIN

Infants and toddlers need a sufficient amount of environmental interaction to display adequate developmental progression. The degree of environmental interaction afforded an infant depends in large measure on the child's ability to exhibit voluntary control of motor functions. For the healthy infant the child's constitution reflects, over time, an evolving neurologic maturation. This results in the attainment of motor milestones at the appropriate time and in the appropriate order. For infants who have experienced neonatal insult, a long-term result may be a delayed or aberrant pattern of neurologic maturation. The result is deficient environmental opportunity, thus contributing to developmental pathology. Hence, motor deficits should be detected at an early age to try to reduce the impact of deviations in motor development through early intervention. Abnormal development of motor skills during early and later infancy may indicate neurologic problems and should be closely monitored. Once the child walks, his or her overall development is enhanced because independent locomotion affords the child the opportunity to explore new environmental territory.

Motor Assessment During Early Infancy

A widely used system for newborn appraisal moments after birth is the Apgar scale (Apgar, 1966). The Apgar scoring system allows a quick yet thorough examination of the newborn's response to the birth process and immediate adaptation to extrauterine life. The infant is assessed 60 seconds after birth and then again at five minutes after birth. Each assessment takes about one minute to administer. In most instances the administration of the Apgar is considered a routine part of the immediate care of the newborn. A large number of studies correlate Apgar scores with a variety of other behavioral measures, including neurologic functioning at later ages. Apgar and James (1962) reviewed data on 27,715 infants. In infants weighing over 1,000 gm there was a highly significant difference in the survival rate of infants whose score was poor (0–3), fair (4–6), and good (7–10). Factors that contribute to infant death contribute to later motor deficits in surviving infants. Numerous other neonatal followup studies have routinely used Apgar scores as a control on the population of infants under investigation. Table 6-16 presents a summary of the Apgar scoring chart. The assessor should become aware of a particular child's Apgar scores as part of the assessment of motor functioning, regardless of age.

An additional instrument widely accepted as a neonatal tool is the *Brazelton Neonatal Behavioral Assessment Scale* (BNBAS) (Brazelton, 1973). The BNBAS is an interactive examination measuring a variety of aspects of infant behavior. Designed for the assessment of neonates (infants

TABLE 6-16. Apgar scoring chart

Sign	Score 0	Score 1	Score 2
Heart rate	Absent	Slow (below 100)	Over 100
Respiratory effort	Absent	Slow, irregular hypoventilation	Good, crying lustily
Muscle tone	Flaccid	Some flexion of extremities	Active motion, well flexed
Reflex irritability	No response	Cry, some motion	Vigorous cry
Color	Blue, pale	Body pink, hands and feet blue	Completely pink

Source: Adapted from V. Apgar (1966). The newborn (APGAR) scoring system: Reflections and advice. *Pediatric Clinics of North America, 13,* 645.

from birth to 1 month of age), the scale measures individual differences at an early age. It may be used as a diagnostic tool for neurologic impairment and as a psychological scale for early individual differences in infants (Tronick and Brazelton, 1975). The scale includes 20 reflex items, 27 behavioral response items, ratings of predominant states during the examination, and a description of self-quieting activities used by the infant.

BNBAS results have been used by some to predict later neonatal ability (Horowitz, Self, and Paden 1971; Tronick and Brazelton, 1975; Brazelton, 1981). The results of the BNBAS provide evidence of cortical control and responsiveness, even in the neonatal period. The neonate's capacity to manage and overcome the physiologic demands of this adjustment period to attend to, to differentiate, and to habituate to the complex stimuli of an examiner's maneuvers may be an important predictor of the baby's future central nervous system (CNS) organization. Several additional instruments designed to assess neurobehavioral integration in the newborn period include the *Albert Einstein Neonatal Neurobehavioral Scale Manual* (Daum, Grellong, and Kirtzberg, 1977), the *Neurological Assessment of Preterm and Fullterm Infant* scale (Dubowitz and Dubowitz, 1981), and the *Longitudinal Neurobehavioral Assessment Procedure for Preterm Infants* (Korner, Schneider, and Forrest, 1983). Als (1985) reports on the predictive ability of the *Assessment of Preterm Infants' Behavior* test. This instrument has shown predictive validity to 9 and 18 months postterm and to performance at 5 years.

Touwen (1976) presented a compilation of criteria for neonatal neurological optimality. This information can be used by the assessor in determining whether an infant is displaying appropriate neurologic behaviors during the early infancy period. An adaptation of the material is presented in Table 6-17.

TABLE 6-17. Criteria for neonatal neurologic optimality

Behavior	Observation
Resting posture	Symmetric; flexion, semiflexion
Facial innervation	Symmetric during rest, movement
Spontaneous motility	Alternating movements
Intensity of spontaneous motility	Medium intensity
Deviant motility	Absent
Fontanelles	Normal range and consistency
Nystagmus	Absent
Knee jerk	Brisk and symmetric
Rooting	Present in four directions
Sucking	Powerful and regular
Palmar grasp	Symmetric; medium intensity
Withdrawal reflex	Present and symmetric
Asymmetric tonic neck reflex	Symmetric if present
Moro threshold reflex	Medium
Spontaneous crawling movements	Present and symmetric
Stepping movements	Present and symmetric
Crying	Normal pitch
State changes	Mild and easily influenced

Source: Adapted from B. Touwen (1976). *Neurological development in infancy*. London: Heineman Medical Books.

The significance of early neurologic assessment for infants was discussed by Prechtl (1983). It is crucial to identify newborns who may have CNS damage due to prenatal or perinatal complications. The examiner should attempt to identify conditions that might be considered risk factors or signs of risk in selecting those infants who have a statistically higher chance of being affected. Unfortunately, sequelae of risk factors are not always clear-cut, since they may vary from death to a multitude of handicaps (e.g., epilepsy, cerebral palsy, mental retardation), minor neurologic signs (e.g., mild paresis, hypotonia, mild dyskinesia), and behavioral disabilities (e.g., reading difficulties, attentional deficits, sleep problems). The question of which infants will be affected and display any of the sequelae specified previously is not easy to answer.

Motor Assessment Following Early Infancy

One way deficient motor development may be detected is to compare an individual child's reflex patterns with normal reflex patterns. Table 6-18

TABLE 6-18. Reflexes and signs during the first year

Reflex	Appears	Disappears
Moro	Birth	4-5 months
Stepping and placing	Newborn	Persists as standing
Positive supporting	Newborn-3 months	Persists voluntarily
Tonic neck	2-3 weeks	4-6 months
Neck righting	4-6 months	Persists voluntarily
Grasp		
Palmar	Birth	3-4 months
Palmar (whole hand)	Persists voluntarily after four months	
Pincer	Persists voluntarily after 6-7 months	

presents an overview of reflexes and signs that should appear during the first year. It is important that the assessor, regardless of primary discipline, become familiar with the normal progression of motor development.

As may be observed, several signs should disappear, and additional signs should appear. A further discussion of these signs should assist the practitioner in better understanding the normal sequence of motor development during the first year. The information to follow should serve as important indexes of nervous system maturation (Weiner, Bresnan, and Levitt, 1982).

The following reflexes and signs disappear:

1. *Moro reflex.* The Moro reflex is a sudden abduction of the arms, extension of the legs, and flexion of the hips when the position of the head is changed abruptly in relationship to the body. The Moro reflex should be present in all normal full-term infants. An indicator of the intactness of the nervous system, it diminishes during the first months of life and usually disappears by 4 to 5 months of age.

2. *Tonic neck reflex.* If the infant is placed in a supine position and the head is turned to one side, the result should be an extension of the arm and leg on that side with flexion of the contralateral arm (fencing posture). It is usually not present in the newborn but appears after two or three weeks. It is most prominent in the second month of life, and infants may assume it spontaneously. An obligate or persistent tonic neck reflex is abnormal. In an obligate or abnormal response the infant maintains the tonic neck posture as long as the head remains turned to one side. A consistently asymmetric tonic neck response may be an early sign of hemiparesis on the side of increased response. The reflex is rarely present after 5 or 6 months

of age. Persistence after this time is abnormal. Sitting is usually impossible until this reflex disappears.

3. *Crossed adductor reflex.* Contraction of both hip adductors when either knee jerk is elicited reflects the crossed adductor reflex. The crossed adductor reflex usually disappears by 7 to 8 months of age. Persistence beyond that time reflects dysfunction.

4. *Babinski response.* The Babinski (extensor plantar) response is usually considered normal until 1 year of age. It is considered abnormal during the first year only if it is repeatedly and easily elicited, asymmetric, or associated with other abnormal signs.

The following reflexes and signs appear:

1. *Neck righting reflex.* If the infant is in a supine position and the head is turned to one side, the infant should turn the neck and trunk to the same side. This appears when the tonic neck reflex disappears (at approximately 4 months of age when the baby begins to roll over). All normal infants have a neck righting reflex by age 8 to 10 months, after which it becomes part of voluntary activity.

2. *Handgrasp.* By 4 to 5 months of age the infant should be able to reach and grasp with the whole hand. Thumb and finger (pincer) grasp begins at 6 to 7 months of age and is present in normal infants by 1 year of age. Transferring objects from one hand to the other begins at 7 to 9 months. A strong preference to use one hand is abnormal before 1 year of age, when the first clear evidence of handedness appears.

3. *Posture in horizontal suspension.* In a test of head control and motor function, infants at 5 months, when held horizontally (parallel to the floor), should begin to hold their head above the horizontal plane.

4. *Parachute reflex.* At approximately 6 to 7 months the infant, when suspended horizontally and plunged downward, should extend the arms to break the fall. This should be well developed by 1 year of age. This is a good measure of upper extremity function; if asymmetric, it may be a sign of hemiparesis.

A concise and easy to understand description of motor development and maturational changes in infancy has been presented by Shirley (1959). Maturational changes are described as a series of advances presented as first-through-fifth-order skills. These advances are not random or haphazard but follow an orderly plan: (1) the baby gains control of the upper trunk, (2) postural control moves downward to include the entire trunk region and, in addition, exhibits activity directed toward locomotion, (3) active and rigorous effort at locomotion is observed, (4) postural control of the entire body becomes complete, and (5) postural control and coordination are combined as the child reaches the goal of walking sometime around 12 months of age. A summary of these stages is presented in Table 6-19. This information can be used by the assessor as a basis for comparison if delayed motor maturation is suspected for an individual child. These milestones reflect median ages, although some variation around these ages may be observed. However, a consistent pattern of deviation from the normal developmental sequence of motor skills should be examined closely, since it may warrant additional referrals for medical-neurologic evaluation.

TABLE 6-19. Median age of acquisition of motor skills

Stage	Median age (wk)
First-order skills	
On stomach — chin up	3.0
On stomach — chest up	9.0
Held erect, stepping	13.0
On back, tense for lifting	15.0
Held erect, knees straight	15.0
Sit on lap, support at lower ribs	18.5
Complete head control	18.5
Second-order skills	
Sit alone momentarily	25.0
On stomach, knee push or swim	25.0
On back rolling	29.0
Held erect, stand firmly with help	29.5
Sit alone 1 minute	31.0
Third-order skills	
On stomach, some progress	37.0
On stomach — scoot backward	39.5
Fourth-order skills	
Stand holding to furniture	42.0
Creep	44.5
Walk when led	45.0
Pull to stand by furniture	47.0
Fifth-order skills	
Stand alone	62.0
Walk alone	64.0

Source: Adapted from M. Shirley (1959). *The first two years: A study of 25 babies.* Minneapolis: University of Minnesota Press.

Categories of Complications

One paradigm that has been proposed to describe common motor abnormalities seen in infants was presented by Ellison (1984). Three categories of abnormalities are included. The first is *cerebral palsy,* which has been defined as nonprogressive, chronic disability characterized by aberrant control of movement and posture appearing early in life. Abnormal movement and posture during infancy are not difficult to detect; however, some infants outgrow this abnormality, most in late infancy and some in preschool years, leaving only a remnant of chronic disability at 7 years of age.

Motor dysfunction in infancy is the second category described by Ellison (1984). This is an umbrella term that refers to four types of dysfunction. It covers abnormalities that remain as well as those that eventually disappear. It differs from cerebral palsy in that the specific muscles involved may be mixed, as may the type of involvement among muscle groups. These four types of dysfunction are characterized by the following:

1. An involvement of all four limbs that differs from that characterized by abnormal tension of muscles (hypertonia). The infant may have hypotonia of the arms and spasticity of the legs or a dyskinetic quality to arm movement and posture and spasticity of the legs.
2. A one-sided movement, generally with more involvement of the arm than of the leg.
3. Bilateral leg involvement (with lesser involvement of the arms), often manifested as some delay or clumsy fine motor control rather than spasticity.
4. A delay in head control, sitting with rounded back, delay in independent sitting, and delay in leg control with delayed pulling to standing, cruising, and independent walking.

The final category described by Ellison is *transient abnormalities of infancy.* Transient abnormalities fall between the abnormal and the normal. These are observations of abnormal function that appear and disappear at different ages of infancy. The recurrent theme is that of neurologic abnormality that disappears by late infancy. This final category poses methodologic problems for the assessor attempting to determine neurologic adequacy in the infant. Knowledge of risk history is important; however, it is certainly not foolproof in predicting later neurologic sequelae. It would be naive to expect a one-to-one relation between early and later neurologic findings. How close the correlation will be depends on a variety of methodologic and biologic factors. Even in light of the transient nature of factors concerning motor functioning in infancy, data exist regarding the correlation between neurologic examination findings and later performance.

Dubowitz et al. (1984) report such data. A cohort of 129 infants at gestational ages of 34 weeks and below were followed at one year to determine neurologic status. Of the 62 infants considered normal at 40 weeks' gestational age, 91 percent were assessed as normal at 1 year. Thirty-nine infants were considered to be abnormal at 40 weeks' gestational age. Of these infants, only 35 percent were considered to be normal at 1 year of age. The authors conclude that infants with a cluster of behaviors (head lag, abnormal tone, trunk hypotonia, miscellaneous deviant neurologic signs) during the neonatal period are more likely to continue to display abnormal neurologic findings at 1 year of age. Table 6-20 presents an adaptation of the criteria described in the Dubowitz et al. study. The criteria presented in Table 6-20 are those used by the authors in determining the infants who, at 40 weeks, were considered to have abnormal neurologic development.

Assessment Tools

A review of the more widely used early childhood assessment tools reveals that many of them pay particular attention to motor functioning. Many of these instruments have subscales or portions that assess motor skills specifically or in the context of overall developmental assessment. Other instruments target motor skills alone.

A widely used scale for the assessment of motor functioning in early childhood is the *Bayley Scales of Infant Development* (Bayley, 1969). The Bayley is designed to provide a tripartite basis for the evaluation of a child's developmental status in the first 30 months of life. The motor scale of the Bayley is designed to provide a measure of the control of the body, coordi-

TABLE 6-20. Criteria for neurologic abnormality at 40 weeks

ABNORMAL

Marked trunk hypotonia plus head lag

Three abnormal signs *

BORDERLINE

Two abnormal signs *

One abnormal * sign plus suboptimal head control

* Abnormal signs include: (1) arm flexor tone greater than leg flexor tone, (2) head control abnormal: poor, differential, (3) increased tremors plus startling, (4) persistently adducted thumb, (5) abnormal Moro reflex (extension only), (6) abnormal eye movement, and (7) irritability.
Source: Adapted from L. Dubowitz et al. (1984). Correlation of neurological assessment in the preterm newborn infant with outcome at 1 year. *Journal of Pediatrics, 105,* 452.

nation of the large muscles, and finer manipulatory skills of the hands and fingers. Because the motor scale is specifically directed toward behaviors reflecting motor coordination and skills, it is not concerned with functions thought of as cognitive (Bayley, 1969, p. 3). Skills thought of as cognitive are specifically assessed as part of the mental scale of the Bayley.

The mental scale is designed to assess sensory-perceptual acuities, discriminations, and the ability to respond to these; the early acquisition of object constancy and memory, learning, and problem solving ability; vocalizations and the beginnings of verbal communication; and early evidence of the ability to form generalizaitons and classifications, which is the basis of abstract thinking (Bayley, 1969, p. 3).

The final portion of the Bayley is known as the infant behavior record (IBR). The IBR is completed after the mental or motor scale of the Bayley has been administered. The IBR helps the administrator assess the nature of the child's social and objective orientations toward the environment as expressed in attitudes, interests, emotions, energy, activity, and tendencies to approach or withdraw from stimulation (Bayley, 1969, p. 4). The Bayley has been widely used as a clinical and research tool to assess children at risk for developmental delay, as a measure of the effectiveness of intervention services, and as a tool to monitor developmental change over time. Overall the Bayley has been shown to be reasonably reliable, with good agreement among examiners (Weiner and Bayley, 1986; Yang, 1979). It has been found to measure child development in a manner consistent with available theories of child development (Yang, 1979).

Examples of instruments that target motor skills alone include the *Peabody Developmental Motor Scales* (Folio and Fewell, 1983) and *A Motor Development Checklist* (Doudlah, 1976). The Peabody provides normative data on a nationwide sample and a thorough assessment of motor development. It consists of a gross and fine motor scale. The gross motor scale contains ten items at each age level and is divided into five categories: reflexes, balance, nonlocomotion, locomotion, and receipt and propulsion of objects. The fine motor scale contains eight items at each age level and is divided into four skill categories: grasping, hand use, eye-hand coordination, and manual dexterity. Each item is scored on a 0- to 2-point scale, with a score of 1 indicating partial success (Palisano and Lydic, 1984). The Peabody takes approximately 20 to 30 minutes per scale to administer and is intended for use with children birth through 83 months of age. No reliability or validity data are available on the *Motor Development Checklist.*

Summary of Motor Domain

Provided there are not threatening interval complications, a normal neonatal neurologic finding has a higher predictive value for later normal motor development. The practitioner must keep in mind, however, that suspect neurologic findings in infancy may not be highly predictive of later motor problems because of the transiency of these behaviors. Unless severe dysfunction is present in the first months of life, the outlook for neuromotor development cannot be reliably ascertained. As the child is followed by the practitioner during the first year, however, a more reliable prognosis of later neuromotor maturation may be determined. The presence of neurologic dysfunction during the first year predicts later minor dysfunction in certain populations of infants. This includes infants who display motor deficits secondary to birth asphyxia and intercranial hemorrhage. Hence, it is imperative that motor development be monitored from the time risk is established. Even in the absence of known risk, those children who fail to display a normal progression of motor maturation should receive regular followup. Regardless of primary discipline, each practitioner should be alert to, and assist in monitoring, the motor development of children from birth to 3 years of age.

COGNITIVE DOMAIN

The term *cognition* has traditionally been used to refer to symbolic and representational thought processes that do not necessarily depend on immediate perceptual input. Since predictable and organized behavior in early infancy does not appear to depend on immediate perceptual input, it has been questioned whether infants can be considered to function cognitively. Cognition cannot be directly observed or measured but is inferred from the behavior of an individual within a specified context. Changes in behavior in similar contexts over time are assumed to reflect changes in cognitive functioning or structuring.

Without doubt, the most comprehensive theory of cognitive development has been put forth by Jean Piaget. In 1952 Piaget declared that the basic principles of cognition and biologic development are the same and that cognition cannot be separated from the organism's total functioning (Piaget, 1952). Piaget indicated that as an organism develops, its conceptual system changes. Hence, the conceptual system consists of organized patterns of reacting to stimuli. These organized patterns are termed *schemata*. Schemata are the cognitive structures of an individual that are used to process incoming sensory information. The first 2 years of life have been termed the sensorimotor stage of development by Piaget. It is during these years that cognitive development is initiated and when schemata are begun.

For example, when an object that a 7-month-old child has shown interest in is completely hidden under a cloth, the infant may not search for it, even though it can be demonstrated that the child has the motor ability to lift the cloth. Several months later, this same infant will actively search for an object hidden in this way (Piaget, 1952). From the change in behavior in the same situation, it is inferred that the cognitive structures (schemata) of the infant have changed so that the child is able to conceive of finding objects that are not immediately visible. It is precisely this type of change that interests assessors concerning how the presence or absence of various behaviors influence judgments regarding cognitive skills in infants and toddlers.

Today, it is generally accepted that a number of skill areas must be considered to assess adequately an infant's cognitive functioning (e.g., object permanence, verbal and gestural imitation). In addition, it appears impossible to obtain an assessment of cognitive functioning without also requiring the child to make use of motor, social, and communication skills. Lewis has described infant-toddler intelligence as "not a general unitary trait, but rather a composite of skills and abilities" (1976, p. 14). Hence, much of what has been previously described in the present chapter has a direct impact on procedures designed to determine cognitive skill level for infants and toddlers.

An attractive paradigm in which to view infant-toddler cognition was presented by McCall (1979). In this paradigm mental performance is viewed as changing as various stages of cognitive development are reached. This view is certainly similar to other views of cognitive growth, particularly Piaget (1952). McCall states that changes in mental behavior serve two functions: the acquisition of information and the disposition of the organism to influence the inanimate and animate environment to which it is exposed. The stages, and the descriptive behaviors within each stage, are presented below.

1. *Newborn stage.* Stage I covers the first 2 months of life, when the infant primarily exercises endogenous, structural behavioral dispositions and selective but basically responsive attention to certain aspects of the environment.

2. *Subjectivity.* The subjective stage stretches from approximately 2 to 7 or 8 months of age. During this stage the world is known by and is indistinguishable from the infant's perceptual-motor and physical action with it. This is complete subjectivity because, in a sense, objects are what the infant does with them. Therefore, the infant acquires information by exploratory behavior, especially that producing some obvious perceptual consequence.

3. *Separation of means from ends.* The onset of the stage of separating means from ends is approximately 8 months of age. At this point infants can distinguish between objects and their actions, but a strong reliance on interaction with objects is needed for the child to really know the object. A more goal-oriented pattern of exploration is observed. Initial attempts at imitation may also be seen at this point.

4. *Entity-entity relations.* At approximately 13 months the infant can appreciate the independence of entities and understand that they carry

their own properties, including the potential to be independent forces in the environment. It is at this point that the infant can see one object in relation to another object without having to act on these objects. This ability enhances information acquisition by permitting consensual vocabulary, a skill requiring the infant to relate a verbal entity to a specific object. The infant can also imitate totally new behaviors not previously seen and not currently in the child's response repertoire.

5. *Symbolic relationships.* At approximately 21 months the child can draw symbolic relationships between entities in which one or more of the entities as well as the relationship itself may be symbolically coded. Sequences of actions can be remembered and imitated, and creative two-word utterances are possible.

The assessor will do well to keep these stages in mind as a further gauge of the change seen over time in the infant's ability to organize his or her world. This is at the heart of cognitive development — namely, the infant's ability to organize and make sense of the environment to which he or she is exposed.

Examples of Assessment Instruments

In the context of infant-toddler cognition as a composite of skills across developmental domains, the assessor must be familiar with what constitutes normal developmental skill mastery across these domains. In the same manner, comprehensive assessment instruments must include behaviors that allow the child an opportunity to display behaviors across domains. Once a wide sampling of behaviors is obtained, the assessor can judge how well an individual child displays behaviors that reflect appropriate cognitive functioning.

One caution is needed at this point. Earlier chapters reinforced the tenuous nature of using cognitive measures obtained early in childhood to predict later cognitive ability. Multiple factors interact in various ways to influence cognition. Hence, results obtained on infant-toddler assessment instruments should be viewed as indicating how the child did on that day and not as reflecting potential. It is only in the presence of serial testing that statements regarding future potential can be made with any certainty.

Instruments used to assess cognitive functioning are, for the most part, based on one of two approaches. These are the traditional psychometric methodology or the more recent developmental theory approach. Each of these approaches can be helpful to the practitioner in assessing current functioning, detecting delayed or abnormal functioning to design an intervention program, or evaluating the effectiveness of an intervention. Two instruments will be discussed to point out the differences between these two approaches to the assessment of cognition in infants and toddlers.

Developmental theory assessment approach. The *Uzgiris-Hunt Ordinal Scales of Psychological Development* represents an approach toward cognitive assessment from the developmental theory framework (Uzgiris and Hunt, 1975). These scales were originally developed to assess the influences of differing environments on early development. Test items were selected to represent an ordinal sequencing of cognitive development within each of six major concept areas: (1) object permanence, (2) means-end relationships, (3) imitation (vocal and gestural), (4) causality, (5) construction of object relations in space, and (6) development of schemes for relating to objects. Although the scales are based on Piagetian theory, they are not designed to assign an infant to a specific sensorimotor stage. Infant performance on the scales does provide a measure of current cognitive functioning. In their original form, the scales provided no norms. As such it was difficult to use the scales to determine if a particular child was functioning significantly below his or her age mates. It is possible, however, to look for differences in rates of development in the six areas mentioned. Dunst (1980) has since provided a strategy enabling the assessor to obtain more standardized data following the administration of the scales. The procedures outlined by Dunst afford the assessor additional insights concerning the child's sensorimotor capabilities and aid in the design of intervention strategies.

Psychometric methodology approach. One of the first instruments to provide a well-standardized methodology for assessing infant mental development was the *Bayley Scales of Infant Development* (Bayley, 1969). The test items included on the Bayley were selected empirically according to their ablity to show an increase in the percentage of children who pass with increasing age. The scale consists of 163 items that are ordered by level of difficulty. These items measure responses to visual and auditory stimuli, manipulation and play with objects, responses involving social interaction, object constancy, simple problem solving, shape discrimination, and receptive and expressive language. Each infant is given only that portion of the scale appropriate for his or her age. The raw score is a function of the total number of items passed and does not give any information about specific items passed or failed. The raw score is converted to a normalized standard score (mental development index, or MDI) that represents how an infant compares to age mates in the standarization sample.

A widely used instrument for the screening of developmental/cognitive development is the *Denver Developmental Screening Test* (DDST). The DDST is designed to quickly identify children likely to have significant delays and distinguish them from children who are developing adequately (Frankenburg, Dodds, Fandal, Kazuk, and Cohrs, 1975). The DDST is a quick, easily administered nontechnical instrument suitable for routine use. However, the DDST is a screening device rather than an in-depth assess-

TABLE 6-21. Denver Developmental Screening Test sample items

Domain	Number of items	Description of items	Sample of behaviors
Personal and social	23	Ability to get along with others	Smiles at 3 months; uses spoon at 14 months
Fine motor and adaptive	30	Uses hands well	Hands together at 2 months; two-block tower at 13 months
Language	21	Ability to hear, understand, and use language	Laughs at 2 months; says "Dada/mama" at 24 months
Gross motor	31	Ability to sit, walk, and run	Rolls over at 3 months; walks well at 12 months

Source: Adapted from W. Frankenburg, J. Dobbs, A. Fandal, E. Kazuk, and M. Cohrs (1975). *Denver Developmental Screening Test: Reference manual.* Boulder, CO: University of Colorado Medical Center.

ment instrument. Table 6-21 presents a sampling of items by age presented on the DDST.

An additional scale designed to assess infants is the *Gesell Developmental Schedules.* The current version of the Gesell, which represents revisions by Knobloch, Stevens, and Malone (1980), expands the ages covered from 1 to 36 months. Originally the schedule was organized to cover four broad groups of behaviors: motor, language, adaptive, and personal social. In the revised schedule fine and gross motor skills are viewed as separate categories. The Gesell has been criticized in the past as having a weak normative base and little empirical evidence of satisfactory reliability and validity. Although not as widely used as in the past, it provided a framework from which subsequent assessment instruments arose.

An additional assessment instrument that has been widely used is the *McCarthy Scales of Children's Abilities* (McCarthy, 1972). This scale is designed for use for children 2½ through 6 years of age. The McCarthy offers a general cognitive index derived from a variety of language and nonlanguage thinking tasks. Cognitive skills are broken down into verbal, perceptual/performance (nonverbal thinking and problem solving), and quantitative (number knowledge and reasoning) indexes. The McCarthy also assesses important noncognitive functions that are reported as a memory index and a motor index. The values obtained on these memory and motor tasks are not combined with other indexes when calculating a general cognitive index. Appendix B lists a variety of assessment instruments designed to determine cognitive level for infants and toddlers. It is up to the assessor to determine the type of instrument that will be used in assessing cognitive functioning during the infant-toddler years.

Summary of Cognitive Domain

Material presented in the preceding section, and in previous chapters, has alluded to the fact that assessment data collected early in infancy are not highly predictive of later cognitive functioning. This should always be kept in mind as assessment activity is initiated. At best the assessor is eliciting a sample of behaviors with which later samples may be compared. It is this type of longitudinal review of developmental progress that affords the practitioner the best hope of accurately judging developmental level.

When considering the cognitive domain, the assessor is dealing with processes that cannot be directly measured but only assumed based on observed behaviors. Although a number of assessment instruments are available, both in depth and screening, it is ultimately the assessor's observational skill and integrating ability that will allow accurate and reliable judgments of cognitive functioning. No assessment instrument is foolproof. No matter how impressive a particular instrument may appear, it is only as good as the person using it. As such infant-toddler assessors should always search for innovative ways to elicit behaviors to which significance may be attached concerning developmental skill mastery.

One such example is reported by Ritter (1988), who reports on data indicating that the time an infant gazes at patterns and faces indicates higher risk for decreased cognitive ability by age 3 years. The procedure presents infants with pairs of images, either faces or abstract designs. One is familiar, and the other is new. The time the infant spends looking is measured. Infants who tend to look at each image in a given pair for about the same time are considered to be at risk for later cognitive deficits.

It is precisely this type of work, and others like it, that will assist the practitioner in arriving at strategies to enhance the monitoring of cognitive progress during the infant-toddler years. The enterprise of infant-toddler assessment has made strong progress; however, much remains to be accomplished.

FAMILY ASSESSMENT

One of the major distinctions between previous legislative initiatives to meet the needs of developmentally disabled children and current mandates is the degree to which the family is recognized as crucial to the success of early intervention activity. Early intervention in the context of the family has become of increasing interest to a great number of health care and mental health professionals.

Three factors account for the increased interest in family issues. First, many avenues of support for families in need are decreasing in availability. Thus, more families are identified as needing support in the presence of the stress associated with family functioning. This stress is made more complicated in the presence of a developmentally delayed child.

Second, there is increasing emphasis on a preventive early intervention focus. Fifteen percent (one out of seven) of the children in the United States have a significant mental or emotional disorder, and yet fewer than one out of five of these disturbed children ever receives any treatment (Heincke, Beckwith, and Thompson, 1988). It is argued that prevention must be promoted as an efficient delivery of services methodology. This may best be accomplished in the family context. Thus, acknowledging the importance of the ecologic context of the at-risk or handicapped child when formulating an intervention plan is vital. Increasingly, early interventionists are recognizing that for intervention plans to be effective, they must be developed with a consideration of the many subsystems that affect the child and the parents (Parke and Tinsley, 1982). In an attempt to emphasize further the importance of the family in provision of early intervention services, Turnbull, Summers, and Brotherson (1983) have made the following statements.

1. Each family is unique based on the infinite variations in personal characteristics and cultural-ideologic styles.
2. The family is an interactional unit whose parts are constantly shifting, with varying degrees of resistance to change.
3. Families must fulfill many functions for each family member.
4. Families pass through developmental and nondevelopmental changes that produce varying amounts of stress affecting all family members (pp. 2-3).

What these points emphasize is that regardless of the structure of early intervention services provided, the family must be considered and incorporated into any attempt to intervene for infants and toddlers at risk or displaying patterns of developmental pathology.

Third, recent federal mandate (P.L. 99-457; see Chapter 1) requires that services delivered to handicapped infants and toddlers be provided in the context of the family. Services to handicapped infants and toddlers under P.L. 99-457 include family training, counseling, and home visits and intervention.

Infants and toddlers with disabilities have the same basic needs as all children as well as specialized needs related to the presence of a disabling condition. Practitioners should be directing effort toward ensuring that the child's needs for stability, permanence, and protection are addressed within the context of the family. Additional programming may then be considered to address those needs that are directly evolved from the effects of a disability on the child.

The presence of a developmentally disabled child in the family, or one at risk of developing disability, must certainly be viewed as a considerable stress factor for the family. At times the stress may become severe enough to precipitate a family crisis. Individual families may cope quite differently with the events related to the child's disabling condition. It is useful to view such families in the light of a crisis intervention model, recognizing the nature and severity of the stress, the family's available coping or management abilities, and the family's perception of the situation. The provision of services to assist families in need must be a primary component of any service delivery system.

Several factors relating to a child's disability may influence the nature and intensity of a family's stress. A discussion of the unique forms that family stress may take is provided by Hughes and Rycus (1983):

1. *The degree and severity of the child's disability.* A chronic (long-term) or severe condition tends to be more stressful than a correctable or milder condition. In general, the more the child's disability limits family functioning and interferes with normal family routine, the greater the degree of family stress that might be expected.

2. *The degree of specialized care required.* Some disabling conditions require special care. Special care is time-consuming and difficult for the family. The child's dependence on others to meet needs can put greater demands (stress) on the family.

3. *Visibility.* A highly visible disability may evoke unusual and unpleasant reactions from others. Parents of children with disabilities are regularly confronted with negative, stereotyped attitudes toward the child that may reinforce feelings that the child is "different."

4. *Influences on family coping ability.* Families respond differently to similar degrees of environmental stress. The way a family may respond depends on several factors. These include the availability of resources to help, past experiences in dealing with stress, additional sources of family stress, and the family's perception of the child's disability.

Service delivery systems designed to meet the needs of handicapped infants and toddlers must address each of the areas mentioned above. Overall goals include reducing stress, providing effective resources and supports in coping, and helping the family achieve a realistic understanding of the situation. It is imperative that the assessor, when directing attention toward family assessment, be aware of these and other sources of stress that a family might experience.

In addition to the need to be familiar with sources of stress, it is also quite important that the assessor be familiar with ways these needs may be

met. Even though the assessor's primary area of emphasis may be outside
the scope of family intervention, a working knowledge of categories of service needs will assist the assessor in formulating recommendations following family assessment activity. Service needs fall into several major
categories (Hughes and Rycus, 1983):

1. *Medical needs.* When the child's disabling condition has a medical or
psychological component, continuing medical care or rehabilitation services are necessary. Many disabling conditions result from complex medical
conditions, and regular medical management is therefore mandatory.

2. *Financial needs.* The special needs of many disabled children create
significant financial stress for families. Even with insurance, the costs of
care and management can become immense. Although financial assistance
programs are available, many families may need help in locating and applying for them.

3. *Educational and developmental services to the child.* In many instances
special activities will be provided by practitioners from a variety of disciplines to reduce the impact of the delay noted. The efficacy of early intervention is without dispute. Hence, the assessor should be alert to the need
for such services following initial evaluation.

4. *Case management and resource linkage.* Part of P.L. 99-457 includes
the provision of one professional to serve as case manager. Thus, a qualified
individual will monitor all services provided the child. This is a significant
help to parents, who can be easily overwhelmed by the array of people and
suggestions made to them.

5. *Respite care.* Respite care refers to child care services given to a handicapped child by someone other than the parents to allow the parents some
relief from the stress associated with caring for the child. The astute
assessor should be alert to indications that the parents need respite and
should assist them in finding appropriate respite services.

6. *Parent education.* Parent education services are directed toward increasing parents' capacity to meet the child's special needs. Without appropriate instruction, parents may not be able to care effectively for their child.

7. *Emotional support or therapeutic counseling.* Family responses to the
presence of a handicapped child range from increased strength and cohe-
sion in working together toward a common goal to painful disruption of
family relationships, grief and anxiety, and inability to function effectively.
Some families may require supportive and therapeutic counseling to help
them understand and resolve problems.

The overall goal of family assessment is to identify the areas of need a
family might have and to move toward recommending appropriate intervention
activities to meet those needs. Early intervention in the family system is
directed at changing parental adaptive and responsive functioning to mini-

mize permanent negative effects on the child. Appropriate family assessment is the starting point in this process.

One possible paradigm for family assessment is provided by Bailey and Simeonsson (1988). In this paradigm five areas of family assessment are suggested: (1) parent-child interaction, (2) family stress and needs, (3) critical events, (4) family roles and supports, and (5) family environments. Although the availability of specific assessment instruments in each of these areas is limited, the assessor can use this paradigm to structure observations made of the family, whether formal or informal techniques are used.

The assessor must be aware of various approaches that may be used when attempting to assess family needs. Although a limited amount of instruments exists, those that are available use basically one of two approaches. Family assessment instruments use either a close-ended or an open-ended approach. It is possible for a combination of these approaches to be used (Westby, 1988). A close-ended approach is one in which the parents must choose from fixed responses provided during the administration of the instrument. The advantages of a close-ended approach are that administration and analysis time are shorter. A disadvantage is that the unique experiences a particular family may have been exposed to might not fit the categories and organizational pattern contained in the close-ended instrument. Examples of close-ended family assessment instruments include the *Family Inventory of Life Events and Changes* (McCubbin, Patterson, and Wilson, 1981) and the *Family Inventory of Resources for Management* (McCubbin, Corneau, and Harkins, 1981).

On the other hand, open-ended instruments use a less structured format and individualize questions to a greater degree. Hence, the experienced assessor is more likely to gain information unique or unusual to an individual family. A disadvantage to the open-ended approach is that assessment and analysis time is substantially greater, and more experience on the examiner's part is needed. An example of an open-ended instrument is the *Home Observation for Measurement of the Environment* (Caldwell and Bradley, 1984). Bailey and Simeonsson (1988) provide a format that combines a close- and open-ended approach to family assessment. The *Family Needs Survey* allows caregivers the opportunity to indicate specific areas in which they feel help is needed or not needed regarding the special needs of the family. An adapted form of the *Family Needs Survey* is presented in Fig. 6-6.

Parent-Child Interaction

Information regarding parent-child interaction was presented earlier in this chapter in the context of providing a comprehensive assessment of language functioning. There are additional aspects of parent-child interaction, however, that can assist the examiner in determining if maladaptive pat-

	DOES NOT NEED HELP	NOT SURE	DEFINITELY NEEDS HELP
Information Needs			
1. I need more information about my child's condition or disability.	1	2	3
2. I need more information about how to handle my child's behavior.	1	2	3
3. I need more information about services my child might need in the future.	1	2	3
Support Needs			
1. I need more friends I can talk to.	1	2	3
2. I need someone in my family I can talk to.	1	2	3
3. I need more time to myself.	1	2	3
Explaining to Others			
1. My spouse needs help in understanding and accepting our child's condition.	1	2	3
2. I need help in explaining my child's condition to other family members.	1	2	3
3. I need help in knowing how to respond when others ask about my child's condition.	1	2	3
Community Services			
1. I need help locating a physician who understands my child's needs and me.	1	2	3
2. I need help locating a day care center or preschool for my child.	1	2	3

(continued)

Figure 6-6. Family needs survey. (From D. Bailey and R. Simeonsson [1988]. *Family assessment in early intervention.* Columbus, OH: Merrill Publishing Co.)

	DOES NOT NEED HELP	NOT SURE	DEFINITELY NEEDS HELP
3. I need help locating babysitters for my child to provide me with respite care.	1	2	3
Financial Needs			
1. I need more help paying for expenses.	1	2	3
2. I need more help getting special equipment.	1	2	3
3. I need more help paying for babysitting or respite care.	1	2	3
Family Functioning			
1. Our family needs help discussing problems and reaching solutions.	1	2	3
2. Our family needs help learning how to support each other during difficult times.	1	2	3
3. Our family needs help deciding on and doing recreational activities.	1	2	3

Figure 6-6 *(continued)*

terns of interaction are present. Current data support the notion that parents of handicapped children, or those at risk of developing a developmental delay, are at greater risk of displaying subsequent maladaptive interactive-parenting behaviors. Table 6-22 presents an outline of adaptive and maladaptive interaction behaviors by age. The material presented in this table can certainly assist the assessor in forming judgments about the presence or potential for faulty parent-child interactional patterns. These may in turn be precursors to later aberrant patterns of parental functioning.

Part of the foundation necessary for developing appropriate patterns of parent-child interaction relate to the manner in which the caregiver perceives the child. Broussard (1979) noted that some mothers make a smooth transition from pregnancy to motherhood and have pride and pleasure in raising their infants; the infants generally thrive. Other mothers lack pride in their infants and display little pleasure in motherhood, although physician observations judged the infants to be biologically intact. Thus, physician and mother looked at the same infant and saw different things. As a

TABLE 6-22. Age-related adaptive and maladaptive parental behaviors

Age (mo)	Behaviors	
	Adaptive	Maladaptive
0–3	Invested, dedicated, protective, comforting	Unavailable, chaotic, dangerous, abusive, hypostimulating or hyperstimulating, dull
2–7	In love, woos infant, multisensory pleasurable involvement	Emotionally distant, aloof, impersonal, ambivalent
3–10	Reads and responds contingently to infant's communications across multiple sensory and affective systems	Ignores or misreads infant's communications; intrusive, preoccupied, depressed
9–24	Admiring of toddler's initiative and autonomy; available, tolerant, firm; follows toddler's leads; helps organize diverse and affective elements	Overly intrusive; fragmented, fearful; abruptly and prematurely separates
18–48	Emotionally available to phase-appropriate regression and dependency needs; reads and responds to and encourages symbolic elaboration across behavioral and emotional domains while fostering reality orientation and internalization of limits	Fearful of or denies phase-appropriate needs; engages child only in concrete modes; misreads or responds noncontingently or nonrealistically to emerging communications; overly permissive or punitive
Over 48	Supports more complex phase and age-appropriate experiential and interpersonal development	Conflicted over child's age-appropriate propensities (competitiveness, growing competence, assertiveness, self-sufficiency)

Source: Adapted from S. Greenspan (1983). Parenting in infancy and early childhood: A developmental structuralist approach to delineating adaptive and maladaptive pattern. In J. Sasserath & R. Hoekelman (Eds.), *Minimizing high risk parenting*. Skillman, NJ: Johnson & Johnson Baby Products.

result of this observation, Broussard (1979) developed the *Neonatal Perception Inventories* (NPI). The NPI is an instrument designed to measure maternal perception of the infant. It may be used as an index of maternal perceptions. Results of the NPI may alert practitioners to areas of parent-child interaction that may lead to later difficulty. The NPI consists of two distinct inventories. The NPI 1 is administered during the immediate post-partum hospital stay (days 1 to 4). The NPI 2 is administered approximately four to six weeks after birth. Each inventory consists of two forms designed to be used together. These are the "average baby" form and the "your baby" form. The behavioral items included in the NPI are crying, spitting, feeding, elimination, sleeping, and predictability. The NPI score is obtained by determining the discrepancy between the mother's ratings of her own infant and the average baby. If a mother rates her baby as better than average, her perception is considered to be positive. If she does not rate her baby as better than average, her perception is considered to be negative. In an effort to test predictive validity, 85 mothers from the original pool of 318 completing the NPI were followed by Broussard and Hartner (1971). Evidence suggested that NPI 1 was not predictive of later child adjustment (4½ years) but that the NPI 2 was predictive of adjustment at 4½ years. Such an instrument can assist the assessor in monitoring the development of appropriate patterns of parent-child interaction and identify at an early stage the potential for maladaptive patterns and perceptions.

An additional instrument that may assist the practitioner in gaining valuable information regarding parent-child interaction is the revised *Infant Temperament Questionnaire* (ITQ) (Carey and McDevitt, 1978). The ITQ is a parent-reported questionnaire used to assess infant temperament between 4 and 8 months of age and to assess the mother's perception of these characteristics. Brewer (1982) suggests that the ITQ is of value in a variety of clinical settings, such as physician offices, well-baby clinics, and infant followup and day care settings. Several additional scales reported by Brewer (toddler temperament scale and middle childhood temperament scale) allow the assessor to follow issues related to temperament and infant-toddler–parent interaction throughout the preschool years.

What these and the previously mentioned instruments provide information on is the degree to which the infant and parents are able to establish a mutually satisfying relationship that leads to optimal patterns of parent-child interaction. The presence of optimal patterns of interaction enhances the probability of the parents' developing appropriate strategies to deal with whatever is involved in the care and parenting of a handicapped infant or toddler. The absence of optimal patterns of interaction demands immediate attention. Early identification of faulty patterns is of the essence, and the practitioner is in the best position to monitor and intervene when appropriate.

Several recent investigations point out the importance of detecting maladaptive patterns of parent-child interaction and of providing appropriate intervention when needed. In one of these investigations a cohort of mothers was randomly assigned to a control group or to a group who received a formal support program designed to aid their adaptation to the transition from hospital to home care of their premature high-risk infants. Positive effects of the program on the mothers' sense of competence, perceived control, and responsiveness were evident for the mothers who had needed the most support. Intervention, when appropriate, appears of benefit to mothers of high-risk infants. The key, however, is early detection of those mothers in need of such intervention (Affleck, Tennen, Rowe, Roscher, and Walker, 1989).

Pinata, Sroufe, and Egeland (1989) pointed out the relationship between maternal sensitivity and maternal experiences of emotional support. In a sample of 135 disadvantaged mothers, greater sensitivity to the infant was related to the mother's experience of emotional support rather than to stressful environmental and child characteristics. Two additional investigations discussed maternal self-efficacy and infant attachment as well as issues regarding developmental changes in preterm infants and the impact of family adjustment (Korner et al., 1989, and Donovan and Leavitt, 1989). Clearly, additional investigations are needed regarding early detection and intervention for those factors affecting the development of optimal maternal-child interaction.

Assessing Family Stress, Needs, Roles, and Supports-Environments

Chapter 2 presented a discussion of various models of causation regarding developmental disabilities. It was suggested that the assessor use a transactional view of causation. That is, the assessor must view the family as being in a state of change at any given point. As such, the child's condition affects the family structure and function, and the family's environment, style, and function affect the child. Hence, family stress, needs, roles and supports, and environments may change at any given time. For intervention to be effective, the assessor must be aware of these changes and make appropriate suggestions in light of them. Although there are some specific assessment instruments to help the assessor monitor these aspects of change in the family, nothing can take the place of an observant and astute professional who assists in monitoring family status.

A helpful paradigm that the assessor may employ in structuring various categories of family assessment is provided by Heincke, Beckwith, and Thompson (1988). Although initially proposed as a strategy to assist the authors in completing a comprehensive review of available literature on early intervention in the family context, it also suggests a theoretical framework that the assessor can employ. It is presented in modified form in Table 6-23. Each of the headings suggested in Table 6-23 can assist in structuring observations made of the family in an attempt to keep abreast of transactional changes in family issues. It is up to the assessor to use this framework effectively.

One well-developed assessment tool that collects data regarding specific parameters within the home that are associated with infant-toddler development is the *Home Observation of the Environment Inventory* (HOME) The HOME was developed by Caldwell and Bradley (1970). Separate in-

TABLE 6-23. Variables affecting family status

ECOLOGY OF THE FAMILY

Nature of health care delivery
Nature of housing and the neighborhood
Quality of nutrition
Financial resources available
Support from family and friends

ROLE CONFIGURATIONS IN THE FAMILY

Teenage pregnancy
Single parent versus nuclear family
Employment status
Division of parental roles in the family

VALUES ASSOCIATED WITH FAMILY FUNCTIONING

Child-rearing goals and procedures

PARENT PERSONALITY

Adaptive-competence
Capacity for relationships
Parent's experience of the marriage
Parent's confidence
Knowledge of parenting and family development

NATURE OF FAMILY INTERACTIONS

Marital interaction
Mother-infant interaction
Father-infant interaction
Mother-father-infant interaction
Teacher-infant interaction
Parent-teacher interaction
Peer-peer interaction

MAJOR AREAS OF CHILD'S DEVELOPMENT
AS FOCUS OR RESULTS OF INTERVENTION

Physical health (e.g., weight loss, illness, other)
Cognition (e.g., attention, overall developmental
  progress or lack of)
Achievement
Socioemotional

Source: Adapted from C. Heincke, C. Beckwith, and A.
Thompson (1988). Early intervention in the family system: A
framework and review. *Infant Mental Health Journal, 9,*
2, 111.

ventories were designed to evaluate children from birth to 3 years and from 3 through 6 years of age. A home visit or day care visit must be scheduled with the primary caregiver at a time when the child is awake. The results of the HOME should provide information regarding strengths and weaknesses of the home environment. Thus, a plan can be formulated to assist families in creating a positive setting for childhood development. The HOME lists six subscales for the 0- to 3-year-old child and seven subscales for the older child. Table 6-24 presents a listing of the subscales. The HOME manual should be consulted for examples of specific behaviors that fall within each subscale.

An assessment instrument that assists the practitioner interested in monitoring the type and degree of family stress and adjustment to critical events is the Holmes and Rahe *Schedule of Recent Events* (Holmes and Rahe, 1967). The purpose of this measure is to quantify life events that require individual adaptation and adjustment. It consists of a list of 42 life events dealing with family constellation, marriage, occupation, economics, residence, group and peer relations, education, religion, recreation, and health. Both positive and negative events are included, since both require adaptation to change. Each item on the list is assigned a weight based on the degree of readjustment thought to be required. The summed weight for the events checked by the individual is the total life change score. In an interesting application of the schedule, Barnard, Eyers, Lobo, and Snyder (1983) report that life change scores were correlated with language scores at 4 years of age. That is, the higher the life change, the poorer the language of a group of 4-year-old children. This information is helpful to the practi-

TABLE 6-24. HOME subscale items for each age group tested

Subscale items (0–3 yr)	Subscale items (3–6 yr)
Mother's emotional and verbal responsivity	Stimulation through toys, games, and reading materials
Avoidance of restriction and punishment	Positive social responsiveness
Organization of physical and temporal environment	Physical environment: safe, clean, and conducive to development
Provision of appropriate play materials	Pride, affection, warmth
Maternal involvement with child	Stimulation of academic behavior
Opportunities for variety in daily stimulation	Modeling and encouragement of social maturity
	Variety of stimulation
	Physical punishment

Source: Adapted from S. Calloway (1982). HOME observation for measurement of the environment. In S. Humenick–Smith (Ed.), *Analysis of current assessment strategies in the health care of young children and childbearing families*. Norwalk, CT: Appleton-Century-Crofts.

tioner interested in monitoring family issues, since at least one aspect of later development appears to be related to life change.

Summary of Family Assessment

Prevention is a central philosophy of activity directed toward infants and toddlers. Although present ability to eliminate all developmental pathology is limited, it is possible to identify early factors within the family system that might serve to worsen the effects of the initial disability. A paradigm that recognizes the interplay between the child, parents, and environment is at the basis of prevention regarding family issues. Increased understanding of the ways in which the child's development can be enhanced by supportive parenting is emerging. Likewise, it is increasingly clear that the child's behavior and developmental progress have a definite impact on parenting and family functioning. What emerges is a significant emphasis on supporting parenting needs beyond the early months and to do all possible within the family system to focus on the positiveness of the parent-child interaction and relationship.

Additional issues must fit into the established assessment-intervention protocols. Assessment data must include information about the parent's perception of their children and the impact of their life situation concerning what they are trying to cope with and the resources available to them. The most useful perspective regarding family assessment during the infant-toddler years is one of maintaining a posture of watchfulness to monitor current difficulties in the interplay of infant, parent, and environment. This surveillance is in the interest of being able to lend guidance and support to parents when they are encountering difficulty. Therefore, infant-toddler and parent assessment should be viewed as a positive orientation toward identifying the strength of the individual child and family as well as helping them to monitor signs of disruption.

SUMMARY

Assessment in this text has been viewed as the use of techniques, either formal or informal, that are designed to gather samples of data on which inferences about developmental adequacy can be made. Throughout this chapter a variety of informal and formal techniques have been presented and discussed regarding the assessment of developmental performance across developmental domains. No single discipline is in a position to provide all that is needed regarding infant-toddler assessment. Within the guidelines of federal mandate, it is imperative that all practitioners work together to provide comprehensive assessment services to the children we serve. What this intimates is that in a very real way we need each other. We need each other to provide balance in the actual provision of assessment activity and in the development of new and innovative techniques to identify and intervene for children displaying developmental pathology. Developing strategies to assist in better working together are not an option but a necessity. The result will be a highly competent and compassionate system of services for handicapped infants and toddlers.

STUDY QUESTIONS

1. Discuss why the assessment of maternal attachment and infant caregiver interaction is important as part of a comprehensive communication assessment.
2. Various reflexes that appear and disappear during the infant-toddler years were presented in this chapter. Identify those reflexes that appear during the child's first year.
3. Both process- and psychometric-oriented cognitive assessment strategies were outlined in this chapter. Describe each, and give an example of an assessment instrument that fits each category.
4. What is the difference between a global and a domain-specific assessment instrument?
5. In assessing family stress, needs, roles, and supports, what specific areas might the assessor be concerned with?

REFERENCES

Affleck, G., Tennen, H., Rowe, J., Roscher, B., & Walker, L. (1989). Effects of formal support on mother's adaptation to the hospital-to-home transition of high risk infants: The benefits and costs of helping. *Child Development, 60,* 488.

Als, H. (1985). Patterns of infant behavior: Analysis of later organizational difficulties? In F. Duffey & N. Gerschwind (Eds.), *Dyslexia: A neuroscientific approach to clinical evaluation.* Austin, TX: PRO-ED.

Als, H. (1977). The newborn communicates. *Journal of Communications, 27,* 2, 66.

Antoniadis, A., Didow, S., Lockhart, S., & Moroge, P. (1984). Screening for early cognitive and communicative behaviors. *Communique, 9,* 14.

Apgar, V. (1966). The newborn (APGAR) scoring system: Reflections and advice. *Pediatric Clinics of North America, 13,* 645.

Apgar, V., & James L. (1962). Further observations on the newborn scoring system. *American Journal of Diseases in Children, 104,* 419.

Avant, P. (1982). A maternal attachment assessment strategy. In S. Humenick-Smith (Ed.), *Analysis of current assessment strategies in the health care of young children and childbearing families.* Norwich, CT: Appleton-Century-Crofts.

Bailey, D., & Simeonsson, R. (1988). *Family assessment in early intervention.* Columbus, OH: Merrill Publishing Co.

Bangs, T. (1975). *Vocabulary comprehension scale.* Allen, TX: DLM Resources.

Barnard, K., Eyers, S., Lobo, M., & Snyder, L. (1983). An ecological paradigm for assessment and intervention. In T. Brazelton & B. Lester (Eds.), *New approaches to developmental screening of infants.* Columbus, OH: Elsevier Science Publishing Co.

Bates, E., Beeghly, M., Bretherton, I., Harris, C., Marchiman, V., McNew, S., O'Connell, B., Reznick, S., Shore, C., Snyder, L., Thal, D., & Volterra, V. (1986). *Early language inventory.* La Jolla, CA: University of California.

Bates, E., Bretherton, I., & Snyder, L. (1987). *From first words to grammar: Individual differences and dissociable mechanisms.* New York: Cambridge University Press.

Bayley, N. (1969). *Bayley scale of infant development.* New York: The Psychological Corporation.

Belsky, J., & Most, R. (1981). From exploration to play: A cross sectional study of infant free play behavior. *Developmental Psychology, 17,* 630.

Bernstein, D., & Tiegerman, E. (1985). *Language and communication disorders in children.* Columbus, OH: Charles E. Merrill.

Brazelton, T. (1981). Behavioral competence of the newborn infant. In G. Avery (Ed.), *Neonatology, pathophysiology and management of the newborn.* Philadelphia: J.B. Lippincott Co.

Brazelton, T. (1973). *Neonatal behavioral assessment scale.* Philadelphia: J.B. Lippincott Co.

Brewer, J. (1982). The revised infant temperament questionnaire. In S. Humenick-Smith (Ed.), *Analysis of current assessment strategies in the health care of young children and childbearing families.* Norwalk, CT: Appleton-Century-Crofts.

Broussard, E. (1979). Assessment of the adaptive potential of the mother-infant system: The neonatal perception inventories. *Seminars in Perinatology, 3,* 91.

Broussard, E., & Hartner, M. (1971). Further considerations regarding maternal perception of the newborn. In J. Hellmuth (Ed.), *Exceptional infant:* Vol. 2. *Studies in abnormalities.* New York: Brunner Mazel.

Bzoch, K., & League, R. (1971). *The receptive-expressive emergent language scale.* Austin, TX: Pro-Ed.

Caldwell, B., & Bradley, R. (1984). Home observation for measurement of the environment (rev. ed.). Little Rock, AK: Center for Child Development, University of Arkansas.

Caldwell, B., & Robert, H. (1970). *Home observation for measurement of the environment.* Little Rock, AR: Center for Child Development, University of Arkansas.

Calloway, S. (1982). HOME observation for measurement of the environment. In S. Humenick-Smith (Ed.), *Analysis of current assessment strategies in the health care of young children and childbearing families.* Norwalk, CT: Appleton-Century-Crofts.

Carey, W., & McDevitt, S. (1978). Revision of the infant temperament questionnaire. *Pediatrics, 61,* 735.

Carrow, E. (1973). *Test of auditory comprehension of language.* Austin, TX: Learning Concepts.

Chapman, R. (1981). Exploring children's communicative intents. In J. Miller (Ed.), *Assessing language production in children: Experimental procedures.* Austin, TX: PRO-ED.

Committee to Study the Prevention of Low Birth Weight. (1985). *Preventing low birth weight.* Washington: Institute of Medicine.

Coplan, J. (1987). *The early language of milestone scale.* Austin, TX: PRO-ED.

Coplan, J. (1985). Evaluation of the child with delayed speech or language. *Pediatric Annals, 14*, 3.

Coplan, J., Gleason, J., Ryan, R., Burke, M., & Williams, M. (1982). Validation of an early language milestone scale in a high risk population. *Pediatrics, 70*, 5.

Dale, P., Bates, E., Reznick, J., & Morisset, C. (1981). The validation of a parent report instrument of child language at 20 months. Unpublished manuscript.

Daum, C., Grellong, B., & Kirtzberg, D. (1977). *The Albert Einstein neonatal neurobehavioral scale manual.* The Bronx, NY: Albert Einstein College of Medicine.

Donovan, W., & Leavitt, L. (1989). Maternal self-efficacy and infant attachment: Integrating physiology, perceptions, and behavior. *Child Development, 60*, 460.

Doudlah, A. (1976). *A motor development checklist.* Madison, WI: Library Information Center, Central Wisconsin Center for the Developmentally Disabled.

Dubowitz, L., & Dubowitz, V. (1981). The neurological assessment of the preterm and fullterm infant. *Clinics in Developmental Medicine, 79*, 146.

Dubowitz, L., Dubowitz, V., Palmer, P., Miller, G., Fawer, C., & Levine, I. (1984). Correlation of neurological assessment in the preterm newborn infant with outcome at 1 year. *Journal of Pediatrics, 105*, 452.

Dunn, L., & Dunn, L. (1981). *Peabody picture vocabulary test* (rev.). Circle Pines, MN: American Guidance Systems.

Dunst, C. (1980). *A clinical and educational manual for use with the Uzgiris and Hunt scales of infant psychological development.* Austin, TX: PRO-ED.

Ellison, P. (1984). Neurological development in the high risk infant. *Clinics in Perinatology, 11*, 1.

Enslein, J., & Fein, C. (1981). Temporal and cross situational stability of children's social and play behavior. *Developmental Psychology, 17*, 760.

Folio, M., & Fewell, R. (1983). *Peabody developmental motor scales and activity cards.* Hingham, MA: Teaching Resources Corporation.

Frankenburg, W., Dodds, J., Fandal, A., Kazuk, E., & Cohrs, M. (1975). *Denver Developmental Screening Test: Reference manual.* Boulder, CO: University of Colorado Medical Center.

Gallagher, T. (1983). Pre-assessment: A procedure for accommodating language use variability. In T. Gallagher & C. Prutting (Eds.), *Pragmatic assessment and intervention issues in language.* Austin, TX: PRO-ED.

Gardner, M. (1979). *Receptive one word picture vocabulary test.* Novato, CA: Academic Therapy Publications.

Gesell, A. (1925). *The mental growth of the preschool child.* New York: Macmillan Publishing Co.

Greenspan, S. (1983). Parenting in infancy and early childhood: A developmental structuralist approach to delineating adaptive and maladaptive patterns. In J. Sasserath & R. Hoekelman (Eds.), *Minimizing high risk parenting.* Skillman, NJ: Johnson & Johnson Baby Products.

Hedrick, D., Prather, E., & Tobin, P. (1975). *Sequenced inventory of communicative development.* Seattle: University of Washington Press.

Heincke, C., Beckwith, C., & Thompson, A. (1988). Early intervention in the family system: A framework and review. *Infant Mental Health Journal, 9*, 2, 111.

High, P., & Gorski, P. (1985). Recording environmental influences on infant development in the intensive care nursery: Womb for improvement. In A. Gottfried & J. Gaiter (Eds.), *Infant stress under intensive care.* Baltimore: University Park Press.

Holmes, T., & Raha, R. (1967). The social readjustment rating scale. *Journal of Psychosomatic Research, 11*, 213.

Horowitz, F., Self, P., & Paden, L. (1971). Newborn and four week retest on a normative population using the Brazelton newborn assessment procedure. Paper presented at the annual meeting of the Society for Research in Child Development, Minneapolis, MN.

Horstmeier, D., & MacDonald, J. (1978). *Environmental language battery.* Columbus, OH: Charles E. Merrill.

Horstmeier, D., & MacDonald, J. (1978). *Environmental prelanguage battery.* New York: The Psychological Corporation.

Hughes, R., & Rycus, J. (1983). *Child welfare services for children with developmental disabilities.* New York: Child Welfare League of America.

Jacobson, C., Starnes, C., & Gasser, V. (1988). An experimental analysis of the generalization of descriptions and praises for mothers of premature infants. *Human Communication, 12,* 3, 23.

Kiernan, L. (1986). Preverbal communication schedule. Unpublished manuscript.

Klaus, M., & Kennel, J. (1976). *Maternal-infant bonding.* St. Louis: The C.V. Mosby Co.

Klein, D., & Briggs, M. (1986). *Observation of communicative interaction. A model program to facilitate positive communication interactions between caregivers and their high risk infants* (DHHS Publication No. MCJ 06351-01-0). Washington, DC: U.S. Government Printing Office.

Knobloch, H., Stevens, F., & Malone, A. (1980). *Manual of developmental diagnosis: The administration of the revised Gesell and Amatruda development and neurologic examination.* New York: Harper & Row.

Korner, A., Schneider, P., & Forrest, T. (1983). Effects of vestibular-proprioceptive stimulation on the neurobehavioral development of preterm infants: A pilot study. *Neuropediatrics, 14,* 170.

Korner, A., Brown, W., Dimiceli, S., Forrest, T., Stevenson, D., Lane, N., & Constantinou, J. (1989). Stable individual differences in developmentally changing, preterm infants: A replicated study. *Child Development, 60,* 502.

Largo, H., & Howard, J. (1979). Developmental progression in play behavior of children between nine and thirty months: Spontaneous play and imitation. *Developmental Medicine and Child Neurology, 21,* 299.

Lee, L. (1974). *Developmental sentence analysis.* Evanston, IL: Northwestern University Press.

Lewis, M. (1976). *Origins of intelligence: Infancy and early childhood.* New York: Plenum Press.

Lowe, M. (1975). Trends in the development of representational play in infants from one to three years: An observational study. *Journal of Child Psychology and Psychiatry, 16,* 33.

MacDonald, J. (1979). *Oliver.* New York: The Psychological Corporation.

Macnamara, J. (1972). Cognitive basis of language learning in infants. *Psychological Review, 79,* 1.

McCall, R. (1979). The development of intellectual functioning in infancy and the prediction of later I.Q. In J. Osofsky (Ed.), *Handbook of infant development.* New York: John Wiley & Sons.

McCarthy, D. (1972). *Manual for the McCarthy scale of children's abilities.* New York: The Psychological Corporation.

McCubbin, H., Corneau, P., & Harkins, B. (1981). Family inventory of resources for management. In H. McCubbin & J. Patterson (Eds.), *Family stress, resources, and coping: Tools for research, education, and clinical intervention.* St. Paul, MN: University of Minnesota.

McCubbin, H., Patterson, J., & Wilson, L. (1981). Family inventory of life events and changes. In H. McCubbin & J. Patterson (Eds.), *Family stress, resources, and coping: Tools for research, education, and clinical intervention.* St. Paul, MN: University of Minnesota.

McCune-Nicolich, L. (1980). *A manual for analyzing free play* (exp. ed.). New Brunswick, NJ: Rutgers University.

McLean, J., & Snyder-McLean, L. (1978). *Transactional approach to early language training*. Columbus, OH: Charles E. Merrill.

Miller, J. (1981). *Assessing language production in children: Experimental procedures*. Austin, TX: PRO-ED.

Miller, L., & Yoder, D. (1982). *Test of grammatical comprehension*. Madison, WI: University of Wisconsin.

Mindes, G. (1982). Social and cognitive aspects of play in young handicapped children. *Topics in Early Childhood Special Education, 2,* 14.

Olson, S., Bates, J., & Bales, K. (1982). Maternal perception of infant toddler behavior: A longitudinal construct validation study. *Infant Behavior and Development, 5,* 397.

Olswang, L., Stoel-Gammons, C., Coggins, T., & Carpenter, R. (1987). *Assessing linguistic behaviors*. Seattle: University of Washington Press.

Owens, R. (1988). *Language development*. Columbus, OH: Charles E. Merrill.

Palisano, R., & Lydic, J. (1984). The Peabody developmental motor scales: An analysis. *Physical and Occupational Therapy Pediatrics, 4,* 69.

Parke, R., & Tinsley, B. (1982). The early environment of the at-risk infant. In D. Bricker (Ed.), *Intervention with at-risk or handicapped infants*. Baltimore: University Park Press.

Paul, R., & Fischer, M. (1985). Sentence comprehension strategies in children with autism and developmental language disorders. Paper presented at the Symposium for Research in Child Language Disorders, Madison, WI.

Piaget, J. (1962). *Play dreams and imitation in childhood*. New York: W.W. Norton Co.

Piaget, J. (1952). *The origins of intelligence in children*. New York: International Universities.

Pinata, R., Sroufe, L., & Egeland, B. (1989). Continuity and discontinuity in maternal sensitivity at 6, 24, and 42 months in a high risk sample. *Child Development, 60,* 481.

Prechtl, H. (1983). Risk factors and the significance of early neurologic assessment. In T. Brazelton & B. Lester (Eds.), *New approaches to developmental screening of infants*. Columbus, OH: Elsevier Science Publishing Co.

Reznick, J. (1982). *The development of perception and lexical categories in the human infant*. Unpublished doctoral dissertation, University of Colorado, Boulder, CO.

Reznick, J., & Goldsmith, L. (1988). Multiple form word production checklist for assessing early language. *Journal of Child Language* (in press).

Ritter, M. (1988). Tests can reveal chances of low IQ by age three. *Appleton* (WI) *Post Crescent*, Aug. 15, 1988.

Rogers, S., Donovan, C., D'Eugenio, D., Brown, S., Lynch, E., Moersch, M., & Schafer, S. (1987). *Early intervention developmental profile*. Ann Arbor: University of Michigan Press.

Rossetti, L. (1986). *High risk infants: Identification, assessment, intervention*. Austin, TX: PRO-ED.

Rowan, L., & Johnson, C. (1988). Screening and assessment. Paper presented at the June 1988 infant and toddler communication assessment and intervention workshop, Minneapolis, MN.

Rubin, K., Maioni, T., & Hornung, M. (1976). Free play behavior in middle and lower-class preschoolers: Parten and Piaget revisited. *Child Development, 47,* 414.

Seibert, J., & Hogan, A. (1982). A model for assessing social and object skills and planning intervention. In D. McClowery (Ed.), *Infant communication and development: Assessment and intervention.* New York: Grune & Stratton.

Shirley, M. (1959). *The first two years: A study of 25 babies.* Minneapolis: University of Minnesota Press.

Smilansky, S. (1968). *The effects of sociodramatic play on disadvantaged preschool children.* New York: John Wiley & Sons.

Sparks, S., Clark, M., Oas, D., & Erickson, R. (1988). Clinical services to infants at risk for communication disorders. Paper presented at the annual convention of the American Speech-Language-Hearing Association, Boston, MA.

Stern, D. (1971). A micro-analysis of the mother-infant interaction. *Journal of the American Academy of Child Psychiatry, 10,* 510.

Stickler, K. (1987). *Guide to analysis of language transcripts.* Eau Claire, WI: Thinking Publications.

Tager-Flusberg, H. (1981). Sentence comprehension in autistic children. *Applied Psycholinguistics, 2,* 5.

Taylor, P., & Hall, B. (1979). Parent-infant bonding and opportunities in a perinatal center. *Seminars in Perinatology, 3,* 73.

Terrell, B., & Schwartz, R. (1988). Object transformation in the play of language impaired children. *Journal of Speech and Hearing Disorders, 53,* 459.

Touwen, B. (1976). *Neurological development in infancy.* London: Heineman Medical Books.

Tronick, E., & Brazelton, T. (1975). Clinical use of the Brazelton neonatal behavioral assessment. In B. Friedlander, G. Sterrit, & G. Kirk (Eds.), *Exceptional infant:* Vol. 3. *Assessment and intervention.* New York: Brunner Mazel.

Turnbull, A., Summers, J., & Brotherson, M. (1983). *Working with families with disabled members: A family systems approach.* Lawrence, KS: University of Kansas Research and Training Center.

Update Pediatrics. (1982). *An assessment tool: The infant scale of communicative intent, 7,* 1.

Uzgiris, I., & Hunt, J. (1975). *Assessment in infancy: Ordinal scales of psychological development.* Champaign, IL: University of Illinois Press.

Walker, L., & Thompson, E. (1982). Mother-infant play interaction scale. In S. Humenick-Smith (Ed.), *Analysis of current assessment strategies in the health care of young children and childbearing families.* Norwich, CT: Appleton-Century-Crofts.

Weatherby, A., & Prizant, B. (1988, November). Toward early detection of communication problems in infants and toddlers. Paper presented at the annual convention of the American Speech-Language-Hearing Association, Boston.

Weatherby, A., & Prizant, B. (1989). *Communication and symbolic behavior scales* (exp. ed.). San Antonio, TX: Special Press Inc.

Weiner, E., & Bayley, N. (1966). The reliability of Bayley's revised scale of mental and motor development during the first year of life. *Child Development, 37,* 39.

Weiner, H., Bresnan, M., & Levitt, L. (1982). *Pediatric neurology.* Baltimore: Williams & Wilkins.

Westby, C. (1988, November). Learning how to ask: Working with families. Paper presented at the annual convention of the American Speech-Language-Hearing Association, Boston.

Westby, C. (1980). Assessment of cognitive and language abilities through play. *Language Speech and Hearing Services in the Schools, 3,* 154.

Wig, E., & Seml, E. (1984). *Language assessment and intervention for the learning disabled.* Columbus, OH: Charles E. Merrill.

Yang, R. (1979). Early infant assessment: An overview. In J. Osofsky (Ed.), *Handbook of infant development.* New York: John Wiley & Sons.

CHAPTER 7

Pulling It All Together

Personnel Training Issues
  Survey Data
  Training Programs

Interdisciplinary Issues
  Audiology
  Early Childhood Special
    Education
  Medicine
  Nursing
  Nutrition
  Occupational Therapy
  Physical Therapy
  Psychology
  Social Work
  Speech-Language Pathology

Initiating Infant-Toddler
Assessment Services

Suggestions for the
Practitioner

The Future
  Developments to Date
  Specific Needs: Increased
    Research

Summary

Study Questions

References

The need for reliable, valid, and timely infant-toddler assessment services is clearly understood by an increasing array of professionals. This is readily evidenced by the proliferation of textbooks, journal articles, convention presentations, and in-service opportunities available in the United States. The emergence of similar activity on an international level is forthcoming as well. Although those in decision-making positions on the local level must still be fully convinced of the benefits of early identification and intervention for impending developmental pathology, efforts are underway to accomplish this. Compared with the status of handicapped individuals a generation ago, a profound change has taken place. A variety of forces have fueled that change and will continue to do so.

What issues must yet be dealt with for the full letter and spirit of P.L. 99-457 to be met? What training needs exist? What personnel are needed? It is only as those currently involved in infant-toddler assessment and intervention work together that these questions and others can be satisfactorily answered.

PERSONNEL TRAINING ISSUES

SURVEY DATA

Data on the status of undergraduate and graduate training programs that provide practicum and classroom exposure to issues related to infant-toddler assessment are not abundant. Clearly, increased information about the status of training programs is needed across academic disciplines. One investigation collected data on the degree of undergraduate and graduate training provided for speech-language pathology students (Crais and Leonard, 1988). The authors conducted a telephone and a mail survey designed to determine the current status of efforts to prepare speech-language pathology students to work with handicapped infants and toddlers and their families and to identify needs for training materials and curricula associated with that effort. The telephone survey involved a detailed interview of 48 speech-language pathology training programs nationally. The programs surveyed reported that the bulk of the classroom hours offered covered issues related to normal and abnormal development and case management. The least amount of classroom exposure was afforded to issues regarding infant developmental assessment, infant intervention, family assessment and intervention, and interdisciplinary team functioning. Forty percent of the graduate programs that participated in the telephone survey reported that clinical experience with handicapped or at-risk infants was required as part of the training program. Thirteen percent of the undergraduate programs surveyed and 33 percent of the graduate programs indicated that clinical experience with the families of handicapped infants was required.

A related question asked during the telephone survey dealt with whether the programs allowed for specialization in the area of infancy. Two percent of the undergraduate and 35 percent of the graduate programs surveyed indicated that this option was available. In those programs that afforded students the opportunity to specialize, the coursework was optional and was taken in addition to regular program requirements. Thirty-nine percent of the undergraduate programs indicated that they did not plan to offer infant specialization opportunities within the next five years. Thirty-one percent of the graduate programs indicated that an infant specialty option would not be offered within the next five years. Overall, the results of this survey point to the need for additional coursework and practicum for speech-language pathology students to meet the need for properly trained personnel to work with infants and toddlers.

An innovative approach toward identifying interdisciplinary training issues in light of federal mandates was taken by the Carolina Institute for Research on Infant Personnel Preparation. In 1987 The Frank Porter Graham Child Development Center at the University of North Carolina at Chapel Hill was awarded a grant from the United States Department of Education to establish an early childhood research institute. The institute focuses on the unique issues associated with preparing professionals from multiple disciplines to work with handicapped infants and toddlers and their families. Several important outcomes have resulted as a result of the data collected during the institute's first year.

The first major activity undertaken by the institute was to determine the current status of infant and family academic content in eight disciplines: nursing, nutrition, occupational therapy, physical therapy, psychology, social work, special education, and speech-language pathology. Information was gathered by survey from selected training institutions representing each discipline. The primary purpose of the survey was to determine, within each discipline, the extent to which all students received direct classroom instruction in key areas related to P.L. 99-457. These areas were (1) normal and atypical infant development, (2) infant assessment and intervention, (3) family assessment and intervention, (4) the interdisciplinary team process, (5) case management, and (6) professional values and ethics. The data collected resulted in the formulation of several broad summary statements (Carolina Institute for Research on Infant Personnel Preparation, 1988). These are presented in modified format below.

1. Considerable variability exists across disciplines in the amount of exposure the average student receives in content related to working with infants, toddlers, and families. Undergraduate content related to infant development ranged from 17 to 49 hours. Graduate content related to working with families ranged from 2.8 to 57.3 hours.

2. Considerable variability exists within disciplines in the amount of exposure the average student gets in content related to working with infants and toddlers and their families.
3. In those instances where infant-related content is provided, the main focus is on normal and atypical infant development. Relatively little instruction related to infant assessment and intervention was reported.
4. Overall, very little time is devoted to family assessment and support, the interdisciplinary team process, case management, or professional values and ethics. These findings are significant in light of the content of P.L. 99-457, which requires service to infants and toddlers within these areas.
5. Overlap and confusion appear to exist between disciplines relative to terminology used by each. Clearly, disciplines are interested in the same topics. However, the terms used within and across disciplines make it difficult to arrive at common levels of understanding.
6. In large measure programs surveyed did not anticipate significant increases in the amount of infant-toddler coverage provided the typical student. In addition, programs did not anticipate creating a special early childhood or pediatric course of study. Even in those disciplines that indicated a future increase in coursework, the increase would be on the graduate level and average only six to eight students per year.
7. The primary areas in which programs indicated that the training material and curricula were needed were family issues and interdisciplinary team functioning. Additional issues identified by programs with respect to the need for materials were aspects of infant-toddler assessment and intervention.
8. Several barriers were identified with respect to increasing infant and family issues in training programs. These were competing program priorities, inconsistency with the institution's mission statement, professional organization requirements, and the lack of sufficiently trained faculty and staff.
9. Options are available in existing programs for practicum experiences with infants and toddlers. In actual practice, however, these experiences are rarely required, and only a few students select them as options.

It appears that regardless of discipline, a significant need exists for materials, resources, and undergraduate and graduate training opportunities in issues dealing with infant-toddler assessment and intervention within the family context. It is clear that training programs must examine current curricula and practicum opportunities to maximize student exposure to handicapped infants and their families. These opportunities must be provided in

a variety of settings and should include day care facilities, hospitals, neonatal intensive care units, developmental evaluation centers, and the home.
Home-based practicum sites were the least used as reported in the Crais
and Leonard data. Yet in the context of P.L. 99-457, a significant setting in
which infant-toddler assessment and intervention services will be provided
is the home. There are notable exceptions, however. A handful of training
institutions do offer students the opportunity to specialize in graduate-level
coursework dealing with infant-toddler issues. These are few and far between, however.

TRAINING PROGRAMS

Two examples of institutions that have targeted degree options dealing with
infant-toddler issues are the infant specialist degree program at Rutgers
University in New Brunswick, N.J., and the training program in psychosocial
intervention with high-risk infants at Brown University in Providence, R.I.

The Rutgers University program is intended for students in speech-language pathology, special education, psychology, physical and occupational
therapy, early childhood education, nursing, and social work. Specific
coursework is offered in infant development, handicapping conditions in
infancy, interdisciplinary assessment issues, and early intervention issues.
The program objective is to train students to work with high-risk infants
and toddlers and their families.

The Brown University program is a federally funded training program
designed to train health care professionals in a psychosocial preventive
intervention model with high-risk infants and their families. The courses
address child development, prevention, and intervention, and clinical
demonstration of intervention strategies and procedures. Health care professionals from many disciplines, including child psychiatry, pediatrics,
obstetrics, psychology, special education, nursing, speech-language pathology, and social work, are eligible to participate. Table 7-1 gives a brief overview of the components of the Brown University program.

Each of these programs represents innovative approaches toward training personnel who are equipped to work with handicapped infants. Although programs of this nature are in short supply, existing coursework in
many training institutions is being modified to include increasing infant-
toddler content.

INTERDISCIPLINARY ISSUES

A second initiative taken by the Carolina Institute was to sponsor a working
conference to address key issues in infant personnel preparation. Nine
leaders in each of ten disciplines participated in a three-day conference in

**TABLE 7-1. Components of the Brown University training
program in psychosocial intervention with high-risk infants**

Overview of normal child development, including familial and cultural
  considerations

Principles of prevention and intervention as they relate to assessment,
  treatment, and developmental outcome for high-risk infants and their families

Neurobehavioral evaluation of term and preterm infants

Neonatal behavioral assessment scale including demonstration, training,
  opportunity for certification, and use in intervention

Strategies for assessing parenting skills and clinical interview techniques

Principles and methods for assessing family functioning, adjustment, and social
  support

Assessment of the social and physical caregiving environment and broader
  socioeconomic considerations

Discharge planning, followup, and liaison with social services, community
  resources, and self-help groups

Washington, DC, in May 1988. The ten disciplines represented in the conference included audiology, medicine, nursing, nutrition, occupational
therapy, physical therapy, psychology, social work, special education, and
speech-language pathology. Each discipline was asked to define its mission
and the major roles it perceived relative to P.L. 99-457 (Table 7-2).

An additional outcome of the Carolina conference dealt with an interdisciplinary evaluation of materials and curricula needs. Each discipline was
asked to identify desired and needed materials and curricula. Although all
the needs identified by each discipline cannot be presented in this context,
a sampling of items is presented in Table 7-3.

A review of the needs mentioned in Table 7-3, and others, clearly point
to three areas: (1) increased materials and curricula regarding intervention
services for the family, (2) case management and team functioning issues,
and (3) infant-toddler assessment strategies, materials, and coursework.
Over time the degree to which these identified needs are met will become evident.

A final product of the working conference, and one that should prove
most valuable as efforts are undertaken to enhance interdisciplinary
functioning, was the identification by each discipline of key concepts they
could offer other disciplines, as well as what each discipline would like
from the others. The information presented below represents a discipline-
by-discipline indication of what each can offer and what each would like
from other disciplines.

TABLE 7-2. Mission statements from the Carolina conference

AUDIOLOGY

To provide and coordinate services to children with auditory handicaps, including detecting the problem and managing any existing communication handicaps

EARLY CHILDHOOD SPECIAL EDUCATION

To ensure that environments for handicapped infants and preschoolers facilitate children's development of social, motor, communication, self-help, cognitive, and behavioral skills and enhance children's self concept, sense of competence and control, and independence

MEDICINE

To assist families in promoting optimal health, growth, and development for their infants and young children by providing health services

NURSING

To diagnose and treat actual and potential human responses to illness; for handicapped infants and preschoolers, this means (1) promoting the highest health and developmental status possible and (2) helping families cope with changes in their lives resulting from the child's handicap

NUTRITION

To maximize the health and nutritional status of infants and preschoolers through developmentally appropriate nutrition services within family and community environments

OCCUPATIONAL THERAPY

To promote children's independence, mastery, and sense of self-worth in their physical, emotional, and psychosocial development; purposeful activity is used to expand the child's functional abilities, such as self-help skills, adaptive behavior and play skills, and sensory, motor, and postural development; these services are designed to help families and other caregivers improve children's functioning in their environment

PHYSICAL THERAPY

To enhance the sensory motor development, neurobehavioral organization, and cardiopulmonary status of handicapped or at-risk infants and preschool children within a family and community context

PSYCHOLOGY

To derive a comprehensive picture of child and family functioning and to identify, implement, or evaluate psychological interventions

SOCIAL WORK

To improve the quality of life for infants and toddlers and their families who are served by P.L. 99-457 through the provision of social work services

SPEECH-LANGUAGE PATHOLOGY

To promote children's communication skills in the context of social interactions with peers and family members, in school, and in the community

Source: Adapted from the Carolina Institute for Research on Infant Personal Preparation (1988). *Proceedings of a working conference*. Unpublished manuscript.

TABLE 7-3. Training and curricula needs identified by discipline

AUDIOLOGY

1. Increased practicum with infants and toddlers
2. Improved technology
3. General curricula update of available materials

EARLY CHILDHOOD SPECIAL EDUCATION

1. Family assessment and development of the individualized family services plan
2. Infant-toddler assessment
3. Techniques and strategies for infant intervention

MEDICINE

1. Detailed survey of current medical education to determine the degree of infant-family content afforded medical students
2. Catalog of available videotapes with descriptive comments
3. Methodology for evaluating teacher effectiveness

NURSING

1. Clearinghouse to disseminate information regarding grant projects
2. Teaching modules for graduate and undergraduate training
3. A listing of competencies needed for nurses working with the 0- to 3-year-old population

NUTRITION

1. Clearinghouse to collect and disseminate materials
2. Computer-assisted self-study curricula

OCCUPATIONAL THERAPY

1. Increased knowledge of how to work within the family system and perform family assessments
2. Increased knowledge of theories and concepts of the interactive (synactive) models of development in working with infants and families
3. Increased understanding of how occupational therapy can best function within the interdisciplinary model

PHYSICAL THERAPY

1. Videotapes of case presentations
2. Curricula dealing with case management, federal laws, and the individualized family service plan
3. Loan library of tapes, computer programs, and assessment tools

SPEECH-LANGUAGE PATHOLOGY

1. Annotated references (disk format) of persons who have special expertise in infant-toddler and family issues
2. Video instruction on team and family issues
3. Video of normal and atypical communication interaction in the family context

AUDIOLOGY

What It Can Offer Other Disciplines

1. Knowledge and skills on identification and assessment of hearing function in infants.
2. Selection and fitting of appropriate sensory prosthetic devices.
3. Information on the relationship between auditory functioning and communication development through multiple modalities.

What It Needs From Other Disciplines

1. Knowledge of overall infant develomental disorders.
2. Family systems theory.

EARLY CHILDHOOD SPECIAL EDUCATION

What It Can Offer Other Disciplines

1. Ability to integrate goals from multiple domains, activity-based intervention.
2. Systems approach to linking assessment, intervention, and evaluation of child and family. Specific attitudes regarding disabilities.

What It Needs From Other Disciplines

1. Knowledge of specialized intervention related to specific disciplines.
2. Detailed information on early development process within specific disciplines.
3. Interagency collaboration.

MEDICINE

What It Can Offer Other Disciplines

1. Sharing medical information regarding conditions, treatment, recognition of abnormal development, when to refer to physicians, medical terminology.
2. Technical skills.
3. A healthy skepticism.

What It Needs From Other Disciplines

1. Family functioning information and assessment of family strengths and needs.
2. Working knowledge of functional skills of other disciplines.
3. Vocabulary of other disciplines.

NURSING

What It Can Offer Other Disciplines

1. Knowledge regarding family and child responses to health care or developmental problems and treatment.
2. Assessment of the child's physical and emotional environment.
3. Coordination of care and services.

What It Needs From Other Disciplines

1. Knowledge of findings from all other disciplines.
2. Exploration of legal and ethical issues from an interdisciplinary standpoint.

NUTRITION

What It Can Offer Other Disciplines

1. Nutritional concepts, understanding, and skills keyed to the needs of all disciplines.

What It Needs From Other Disciplines

1. Unique contributions of each discipline in understanding the child and family.
2. Referral criteria for each discipline.
3. Priorities and methods of integrating care into a total intervention plan.

OCCUPATIONAL THERAPY

What It Can Offer Other Disciplines

1. Knowledge of scope of occupational therapy services. When to refer and to seek consultation.

2. Awareness of the impact of sensory training on adaptive functioning.
3. Availability and use of devices and methods to adapt environments.

What It Needs From Other Disciplines

1. Knowledge and awareness of scope of services provided by other disciplines.
2. Knowledge of family systems and dynamics.
3. Service coordination and case management.

PHYSICAL THERAPY

What It Can Offer Other Disciplines

1. Criteria for discriminating normal versus abnormal movement.
2. Knowledge of positioning and handling of infants.

What It Needs From Other Disciplines

1. Greater understanding of family systems therapy.
2. Effective means of communicating with other disciplines.

PSYCHOLOGY

What It Can Offer Other Disciplines

1. Use of empirical approach to practice.
2. Grounding in developmental theory.
3. Appreciation of ecologic framework.

What It Needs From Other Disciplines

1. Knowledge of impact of specific conditions on developmental needs.
2. Increased knowledge of more effective collaboration with other disciplines.

SOCIAL WORK

What It Can Offer Other Disciplines

1. Understanding of impact on families of handicapped children.

2. Knowledge of engaging and working with families from a family systems perspective.
3. Knowledge regarding impact of multicultural diversity and socio-economic factors on family functioning.

What It Needs From Other Disciplines

1. Knowledge of medical conditions and treatment.
2. Knowledge of impact of specific conditions on developmental needs.
3. Knowledge of specific criteria for referral and to develop more effective collaboration with other disciplines.

SPEECH-LANGUAGE PATHOLOGY

What It Can Offer Other Disciplines

1. Detailed knowledge of early communication development.
2. Knowledge of relationship between communication and other developmental domains.
3. Knowledge of family interactions supporting communication of infants.

What It Needs From Other Disciplines

1. Strategies for promoting optimal child performance across developmental domains.
2. Strategies for working effectively with families and community agencies.
3. Strategies to develop more effective collaboration with other disciplines, including referral criteria and terminology used within each discipline.

Data such as these should serve as a blueprint for more effective training within and across disciplines. It is anticipated that the outcome of the Carolina conference will serve to direct the development of curricula, personnel training, and materials for years to come. What emerged from the conference should serve as a working paper from which a variety of future efforts will spring.

INITIATING INFANT-TODDLER ASSESSMENT SERVICES

Although one of the main results of P.L. 99-457 will be to expand the availability of infant-toddler assessment activity, practitioners across disciplines should not lose sight of the role that can be played in serving as an advocate for initiating such services. Regardless of the setting in which the practitioner is employed, the public, colleagues, and those in decision-making positions must be educated. How might the practitioner better serve in an advocacy role regarding the initiation of infant-toddler assessment activity?

One of the first factors that should be considered regarding initiating infant-toddler assessment activity is the particular setting in which the services will be provided. It is imperative that the practitioner employed in a public education setting be familiar with the letter and spirit of federal mandate governing services to children birth through 3 years of age. In addition, individual state variations may exist regarding services to handicapped preschool children. The practitioner should be familiar with these as well, since many states distinguish between mandatory and permissive services. In a situation such as this, the practitioner must assess the need in the community, as well as the local public education agency's willingness, to provide services to children below the mandated ages.

If the need is present, the practitioner should begin to educate those in decision-making positions. The unique needs of handicapped infants and toddlers, the benefits of early identification, and the efficacy of early intervention from a humanitarian and cost-effective standpoint can all be stressed. One source of support that the practitioner should not overlook is parents. Chapter 1 pointed out that in many instances parent groups provided the initial impetus for what evolved into legislation to assist the handicapped. Grass roots efforts can prove quite potent in influencing those in decision-making positions on the local level.

For the practitioner employed in a medical setting, the process of initiating assessment services is similar. Although the number of intensive care nurseries has expanded rapidly in the past decade, unfortunately the presence of systematic assessment and developmental followup programs has not kept pace. It is entirely possible that a practitioner might be employed in a medical setting that contains an intensive care nursery but does not provide developmental followup for infants once they leave the hospital. Several suggestions can be made for the practitioner in such a setting. Once again, the key concept is soliciting support from those in decision-making positions. Pointing out the need for close monitoring of developmental progress as part of a comprehensive child care philosophy is one place to start. Pointing out the efficacy of early intervention, and the need for assessment as part of early intervention, is imperative.

Laney (1985) described a strategy designed to alert physicians and others to the benefits of early identification of developmental pathology. The strategy contains two basic parts with several steps under each. The first major step is gaining access to decision makers and facilitating their awareness of the unique needs of handicapped infants and their families. Gaining access is geared toward both individuals and service delivery systems already in operation. Practitioners in a medical setting should be alert to opportunities to gain access of this nature. Gaining access to service delivery systems that currently do not serve infants and toddlers may involve efforts directed toward well baby clinics, state institutions that serve developmentally delayed persons, and any format in which the parent is asking the health care system for assistance regarding child development issues.

Once needed access is gained, the goal is to facilitate overall awareness of the unique needs of handicapped infants and toddlers and the benefits of early identification. Visits to physicians' offices, lecturing to medical students, participating in pediatric rounds, involvement in staffings in the intensive care nursery, and providing printed material may all prove helpful. Up to 75 percent of pediatricians do not systematically evaluate the developmental performance of their patients (Shonkoff, Dworkin, and Leviton, 1979). Time constraints and lack of awareness and training contribute to this. The practitioner may suggest that a regular schedule of developmental assessments be established for patients for whom skill acquisition is in doubt. Consistent efforts reap long-range benefits from persons in a position to influence the initiation of services to infants and toddlers.

One additional activity is suggested for practitioners interested in creating momentum for initiating infant-toddler assessment activity. Each state is mandated to have in operation a state developmental disabilities council. The overall mission of state councils is to plan, advocate for, and advise on the needs of the developmentally delayed population within the state. Practitioners would be wise to alert themselves to the workings of the councils in their states. Although councils use their allocated funds differently, many councils award grants to persons or agencies geared toward initiating new avenues of service to the developmentally delayed in that state.

SUGGESTIONS FOR THE PRACTITIONER

The information to follow is designed to alert practitioners from all disciplines addressed in this text to a variety of steps that may be taken to enhance service provision to infants and toddlers. Legislators have done their part through the passage of P.L. 99-457. It is now up to the practitioner to demonstrate the same degree of energy and cooperation in making the full intent of the law a reality. Regardless of primary discipline, the suggestions to follow should assist in that process. These suggestions are adapted from Dublinski (1988).

ACQUIRE NEEDED SKILLS

Information presented earlier in this chapter pointed out the degree to which training institutions are not adequately equipping professionals to work with infants and their families. For the professional already working with infants and toddlers, the question arises on where needed skills and training were acquired. In large measure practitioners have had to equip themselves through in-service opportunities and other means. This is not necessarily a drawback, however. Hence, the activities are born of necessity and usually tend to be clinical and applied.

Discipline-specific needs indicated at the Carolina conference demonstrate the degree to which practitioners already in this field need continued input from an interdisciplinary standpoint. The infant-toddler assessor is encouraged to take advantage of all opportunities possible to sharpen clinical skills and expand one's knowledge bases on issues dealing with infant-toddler assessment and related topics.

JOIN STATE INTERAGENCY COUNCIL

As pointed out in Chapter 1, P.L. 99-457 requires the establishment, in each state, of an interagency council to oversee the implementation of the law. The law itself dictates the makeup of the interagency council. Members are appointed by the governor. One effective means available to practitioners of assisting in the full implementation of service to infants and toddlers is to secure membership on the interagency council. If membership on the council is not possible, at the very least practitioners should be aware of who is serving on the council.

In addition, practitioners are encouraged to become familiar with the issues in each state that the council is concerned with at any given time. Substantial issues will be dealt with by the council. Each discipline involved with infants and toddlers and their families should make it a point to guarantee that issues related to their prospective discipline are understood and adequately dealt with by the interagency council. To not be heard is to risk that a full continuum of services may not be afforded handicapped infants and toddlers.

ASSIST IN DEVELOPING STATE DEFINITION OF DEVELOPMENTAL DISABILITY

P.L. 99-457 requires that each state develop its own definition of *developmental disability*. Practitioners must be involved in formulating such definitions. The definitions must be comprehensive enough to cover all developmental domains and thus represent sufficient input from all disciplines involved in service provision to infants and toddlers and their families. The definition agreed on within each state will dictate who is eligible for services for years to come. Thus, the process must be a well-conceived, comprehensive one. Also, issues dealing with service eligibility for infants and toddlers considered to be at risk for developmental disability should be included in the state-adopted definition of developmental disability. This represents an area in which practitioners can provide invaluable input to the interagency council in establishing a service delivery system that ensures appropriate early assessment and intervention services for as broad a constituency of eligible children as possible.

PROMOTE EQUAL REPRESENTATION OF ALL DISCIPLINES ON STATEWIDE CHILD FIND SYSTEMS

Each state is required by law to institute specific procedures for finding infants and toddlers in need of early assessment and intervention services. Thus, states must develop child find systems. There is some latitude on how individual states will develop and implement child find systems. It is quite important that all disciplines provide input regarding the policies implemented in each state to find infants and toddlers in need of services. This might include assisting in identifying assessment procedures and materials used to determine if a developmental delay is present or in identifying procedures and criteria for determining risk status. The entire service delivery system in a given state will only be as effective as the state's procedures in identifying and finding children in need of services. A broad representation of disciplines is encouraged to guarantee an accurate and reliable child find system in each state.

EDUCATE THE PUBLIC

An important part of ensuring that a full spectrum of services is available, and that all eligible infants and toddlers are identified, is educating consumers in each state. Persons from a variety of backgrounds may be in a position to make the initial referral for assessment and intervention services. Most important, parents must be informed of the availability of services, how to access services, and who to contact if they have concerns regarding their child. All aspects of the service delivery system must be included in public awareness activities.

As the general public becomes more aware of the unique needs of handicapped children and their families, increased acceptance will ensue. This has taken place in large measure regarding other groups of handicapped persons. Support groups, parent groups, local legislation (e.g., reserved parking for the handicapped), and other efforts attest to the effect of educating the general public about the unique needs of handicapped persons. There is no reason to suspect that this same degree of public understanding will not result as public awareness of the needs of handicapped infants and toddlers increases.

BE INCLUDED IN STATE CENTRAL DIRECTORY

Each state is required to compile a statewide directory of service delivery institutions and practitioners who meet minimum requirements to provide services under P.L. 99-457. Practitioners are encouraged to ensure that their name or agency is included on the central directory listing. As the references on the central directory grow, practitioners should avail themselves of the list. It will assist in making referrals and in gaining access to other professionals who share similar interests in providing services to infants and toddlers.

BE AWARE OF THE LEAD AGENCY

Each state is required to designate a lead agency. The lead agency is charged with overseeing all activities provided under P.L. 99-457. The lead agency may not be within the state department of education. Lead agencies that have already been designated in states include departments of social services, education, health and human services, developmental disabilities, mental health, and welfare. In some instances the interagency council will serve as the lead agency. Practitioners are encouraged to be aware of the lead agency in their respective state and also to be aware of the contact person. Effective input must be directed toward the appropriate individuals within the lead agency. Thus, familiarity with appropriate persons is essential. Table 7-4 identifies lead agency designations by state.

BE AWARE OF PERSONNEL DEVELOPMENT

It is imperative that in-service activities be provided within each state to guarantee high-quality services to infants and toddlers. Hence, the law requires that a comprehensive system of personnel development be instituted within each state. Practitioners should be aware of who is overseeing this system. Specifically, the personnel development system should include representation from all disciplines, since interdisciplinary provision of services depends on sufficient continuing education within and across disciplinary boundaries. Individual practitioners may elect to be part of the personnel development activities within each state. For personnel devel-

TABLE 7-4. State-by-state lead agency designation by department

State	Agency	State	Agency
Alabama	Education	Nevada	Human Resources
Alaska	Health and Social Services	New Hampshire	Education
		New Jersey	Education
Arizona	Economic Security – Developmental Disabilities	New Mexico	Health and Environment
		New York	Health
Arkansas	Human Services	North Carolina	Human Resources
California	Developmental Services	North Dakota	Human Services
Colorado	Education	Ohio	Health
Connecticut	Education	Oklahoma	Education
Delaware	Education	Oregon	Mental Health Program for Developmental Disability
District of Columbia	Human Services		
Florida	Education	Pennsylvania	Public Welfare
Georgia	Human Resources	Rhode Island	Interagency Coordinating Council
Hawaii	Health		
Idaho	Health and Welfare		
Illinois	Education	South Carolina	Health and Environmental Control
Indiana	Mental Health		
Iowa	Education	South Dakota	Education and Cultural Affairs
Kansas	Health and Environment	Tennessee	Education
Kentucky	Human Resources	Texas	Interdisciplinary Agency on Early Childhood Intervention
Louisiana	Education		
Maine	Interagency Department Committee		
		Utah	Health
Maryland	Office of Children and Youth	Vermont	Education
		Virginia	Mental Health/ Mental Retardation
Massachusetts	Public Health		
Michigan	Education	Washington	Social and Health Services
Minnesota	Education		
Mississippi	Health	West Virginia	Health
Missouri	Education	Wisconsin	Health and Social Services
Montana	Developmental Disabilities		
		Wyoming	Health and Human Services
Nebraska	Education		

Source: Adapted from the National Association of State Directors of Special Education (1987). Washington, DC: Unpublished manuscript.

opment to achieve its desired goal — namely, the equipping of profession-als across disciplines to provide high quality services — all practitioners who have been working with infants and toddlers and their families should be willing to assist in whatever way possible.

BE INVOLVED IN CONTRACTUAL ARRANGEMENTS

The actual services provided to infants and toddlers and their families may be provided by public institutions or private practice agencies or practitioners. Policies must be established in each state to govern contracting for needed services. Practitioners are encouraged to be involved in formulating policies governing contracting of services. These issues include fees, reimbursement, qualified personnel, and quality assurance.

HELP ENSURE THAT PROVIDERS ARE QUALIFIED

The law specifically states that services must be provided by qualified personnel within each discipline. Each state must develop guidelines for monitoring and ensuring that only qualified personnel are providing services. The lead agency and interagency council need input from all disciplines regarding minimum standards for service providers. Procedures must also be developed for situations in which standards are violated. Safeguards for the children and families served necessitate that only qualified personnel be involved in service provision.

SUPPORT INTERDISCIPLINARY COOPERATION

The letter and spirit of P.L. 99-457 includes interdisciplinary delivery of services. This will only become a reality as disciplines cooperate, learn more about each other, and work side by side in serving handicapped infants and toddlers and their families. This can only happen on a person-by-person basis. Hence, each practitioner is encouraged to examine his or her individual understanding of and level of comfort with what is involved in interdisciplinary service delivery. Disciplinary boundaries and controls must be examined. That is not to say that disciplines should lose sight of the unique contributions each can make. Rather, a full realization of the input from other disciplines must be fully appreciated and implemented. In a very real sense, we need each other. As this is fully realized and acted on, enhanced interdisciplinary service delivery will result.

THE FUTURE

DEVELOPMENTS TO DATE

A variety of forces have interacted in an efficacious manner to enhance the prospects for infants and toddlers who display developmental pathology, or who are at risk of doing so. Practitioners currently working with this unique population of clients can readily attest to the benefits seen in the longitudinal outcome of infants and toddlers and families identified early as needing intervention.

The full impact of intervention provided at an early age is not yet known, but it can be assumed to be substantial. Professionals from a host of disciplines are gearing up to better meet the needs of handicapped infants and toddlers. What emerges is a picture of a handful of pioneering professionals who stood by their initial clinical intuition that service to infants and toddlers was worth the effort. Current practitioners are indebted to those who in a large measure set the course before us.

SPECIFIC NEEDS: INCREASED RESEARCH

What lies ahead regarding needs and future avenues of service to handicapped infants and toddlers? Information presented earlier in this chapter outlined what individual disciplines perceived as being their needs. In large measure current needs relate to increased preservice training programs, increased in-service training opportunities, greater availability of tests, innovative assessment procedures, and information dealing with interdisciplinary team functioning. Substantial efforts are already underway in these areas and others. The discussion to follow highlights only a few of the perceived needs for the future.

Past research activity has provided a solid base for many decisions on infant-toddler assessment and intervention. Additional research is needed in several areas of infant-toddler assessment.

Relationship Between Neonatal Factors and Later Developmental Performance

The impact of specific neonatal conditions on later developmental skill acquisition requires additional investigation. The relationship between various neonatal insults and later development is understood only in that a correlation is acknowledged. The nature of the relationship is largely unknown. This has implications for the assessor and intervenor. If atypical development, secondary to neonatal complications, is better understood, more effective identification and assessment and intervention strategies may be developed.

New and Innovative Assessment Strategies

New and innovative infant-toddler assessment strategies are needed. It is no longer acceptable to give a test to see how a child is doing. The assessor must be familiar with existing test materials and strategies but also be willing to rely on experience gained through varied clinical opportunities. How might this experience be quantified, or at least put in a format that makes its application available to large numbers of assessors? This is not an easy question to answer. A combination of experience and strong academic preparation would appear to be the best place to start in ensuring high-quality assessment practices.

In addition, the behaviors that traditional tests put so much emphasis on regarding developmental adequacy have never been subjected to systematic investigation. What does eye tracking indicate? What might a lack of interest in environmental stimulation indicate? New paradigms of assessment are emerging that view many nontraditional behaviors as quite important in overall assessment within and across developmental domains. Also, how do limitations in one developmental area affect performance in other domains? Is there such a thing as normal atypical development? What separates it from abnormal atypical development? A variety of researchers, in an interdisciplinary context, are addressing these and additional issues. The outcome will be new and innovative assessment strategies, techniques, and instruments that will better assist the practitioner in identifying developmental pathology at an early age.

Family Focused Assessment

Significant additions are needed in materials and strategies for the effective assessment of family functioning. All services delivered must be within the family context. Thus, professionals from across disciplines need greater familiarity with family issues. It is anticipated that in the years ahead substantial advances and refinements will take place concerning the accurate assessment of family functioning as well as the provision of appropriate intervention within the family context.

Longitudinal Followup

Enhanced longitudinal data regarding the developmental outcome of handicapped or at-risk children will naturally result from more effective and reliable assessment strategies. One additional result will be a greater ability to demonstrate the efficacy of early intervention, treatment paradigms, varying curriculum, and team functioning models.

SUMMARY

All that will ultimately be involved in the implementation of quality services to handicapped infants and toddlers is not fully known. Will a new category of professionals emerge? Will assessment techniques and subsequent intervention strategies evolve rapidly? What will be the overall cost and impact on society of early identification and intervention on a large scale? These questions can only be answered in time and as an interdisciplinary approach toward assessment and intervention is established. What is clear, however, is that an exciting and unique set of circumstances exists for the practitioner interested in delivering services to handicapped infants and toddlers and their families. The challenge for professionals across disciplines is to be creative and energetic in ensuring a high quality of services. Parents, administrators, legislators, practitioners from all disciplines, and, most important, infants and toddlers and their families will benefit immeasurably from these efforts.

STUDY QUESTIONS

1. How well are existing training programs across disciplines doing in preparing students to work with infants and toddlers and their families?
2. What are some of the interdisciplinary issues that must be dealt with before effective assessment and intervention activity can take place?
3. What are some of the specific steps of action the practitioner might take in ensuring appropriate implementation of P.L. 99-457?
4. Increased research activity in several areas is needed regarding infant-toddler assessment. What are some of these needed areas of research?
5. What are some of the steps that the practitioner might employ in initiating infant-toddler assessment in situations in which none currently exists?

REFERENCES

Carolina Institute for Research on Infant Personnel Preparation. (1988). *Proceedings of a working conference.* Unpublished manuscript.

Crais, E., & Leonard, C. (1988). P.L. 99:457: Graduate training programs: Current practices. Paper presented at the annual convention of the American Speech-Language-Hearing Association, Boston: November.

Dublinski, S. (1988). Legislation: Infants and toddlers with handicaps. Paper presented at the Infants and Toddlers Communication Assessment and Intervention Conference, Minneapolis, MN: July.

Laney, M. (1985). Communication screening and assessment in pediatric populations. Paper presented at the annual convention of the American Speech-Language-Hearing Association, Washington, DC: November.

National Association of State Directors of Special Education. (1987). Washington, DC: Unpublished manuscript.

Shonkoff, J., Dworkin, P., & Leviton, A. (1979). Primary case approaches to developmental disabilities. *Pediatrics, 64,* 506.

APPENDIX A

Sample Questionnaires

SAMPLE 1

PARENTS' QUESTIONNAIRE

Child's full name _____ Birth date _____ Age ____

Home address _____

Home telephone number _____

Child's school _____ Teacher _____

Type of classroom _____

Present home placement of child (check appropriate bracket)

	Column A Adult with whom child is living	**Column B** Other adults (outside home) close to child
Natural mother	( ) _____	( ) _____
Natural father	( ) _____	( ) _____
Stepmother	( ) _____	( ) _____
Stepfather	( ) _____	( ) _____
Adoptive mother	( ) _____	( ) _____
Adoptive father	( ) _____	( ) _____
Foster mother	( ) _____	( ) _____
Foster father	( ) _____	( ) _____
Other	( ) _____	( ) _____

Place the number 1 or 2 next to each check in column A and provide the following information about each person:

1. Name _____ Occupation _____ Age ____

   Business name _____ Address _____

   Business telephone number _____

2. Name _____ Occupation _____ Age ____

   Business name _____ Address _____

   Business telephone number _____

Place the number 3 next to the person checked in column B who is most involved with the child and provide the following information:

3. Name _____ Home address _____

   Occupation _____ Age____ Business telephone number _____

SOURCE OF REFERRAL

Name _____ Address _____

Telephone number _____

Reason for referral (brief summary of main problem) _____

_____

_____

HISTORY OF PREGNANCY, DELIVERY, POSTDELIVERY

Pregnancy: Complications

Excessive vomiting _____ Hospitalization required _____

Excessive staining or blood loss _____

Threatened miscarriage _____

Infections during pregnancy _____

Toxemia _____

Surgeries (specify) _____

Other illnesses (specify) _____

Smoking during pregnancy _____ Average number of cigarettes per day _____

Alcoholic consumption during pregnancy _____

Describe if more than an occasional drink _____

Duration of pregnancy _____ Weeks _____

Delivery:

Hospital _____ Physician _____

Address _____ Address _____

Type of labor: Spontaneous _____ Induced _____

Forceps: High _____ Mid _____ Low _____

Duration of labor: _____ hours

Type of delivery: Normal _____ Breech _____ Cesarean _____

Complications:

Cord around neck _____

Cord presented first _____

Hemorrhage _____

Infant injured during delivery (specify) _____

Other (specify) _____

Birth weight _____ Appropriate _____ Small _____

Post Delivery Period: (while in hospital)

Respiration: Breathing on own after birth

    Immediate _____ Delayed (how long) _____

Cry: Immediate _____ Delayed (how long) _____

Mucus accumulation _____

Apgar score (if known) _____

Jaundice _____

Rh factor _____

Cyanosis (turned blue) _____

Incubator care _____ Number of days _____

Ability to suck: Strong _____ Weak _____

Infection (specify) _____

Vomiting _____ Diarrhea _____ How long _____

Birth defects (specify) _____

Total number of days baby was in hospital _____

Was baby breast-fed _____ bottle-fed _____

Age at which child was weaned to cup _____

PHYSICAL AND SOCIAL DEVELOPMENT

Infancy-Toddler Period:

Were any of the following present, to a noticeable degree, during the first few years of life? If so, describe.

Did not enjoy cuddling _____

Was not calmed by being held or stroked _____

Colic _____

Excessively restless _____

Excessively passive _____

Little sleep because of easy arousal _____

Frequent head banging _____

Constantly into everything _____

Too many accidents compared with other children _____

If you can recall, record the age at which the child reached the following developmental milestones. If you cannot recall, check item at right.

I do not recall exactly, but to the best of my recollection it occurred:

	Age	Early	Normal	Late
Head held up alone				
Sat alone				
Crawled				
Stood without support				
Walked alone				
Fed self with spoon				
Fed self completely				
Spoke first words				
Used one- or two-word phrases				
Spoke in sentences				
Bowel trained day				
Bowel trained night				
Bladder trained day				
Bladder trained night				
Rode tricycle				
Rode bicycle				
Buttoned clothes				
Tied shoes				
Named colors				

Coordination:

Rate your child on the following skills compared with other children the same age.

	Good	Average	Poor		Good	Average	Poor
Walking				Buttoning			
Running				Writing			
Throwing				Athletic			
Catching				ability			

COMPREHENSION AND UNDERSTANDING

Do you consider your child to understand directions and situations as well as other children the same age? _____ If not, describe _____

_____

How would you rate your child's overall level of intelligence compared with other children?   Below average _____ Average _____ Above average _____

SPEECH AND LANGUAGE DEVELOPMENT

Before 1 year of age did your child babble, coo, squeal? _____

Did your child's vocal behavior seem normal to you? _____
If not, describe _____

Did your child ever acquire one or two words and then go for a long time before acquiring others? _____

Did your child keep adding words once he or she began to talk? _____

Did speech learning ever seem to stop for a time? If so, describe _____

_____

_____

At what age did your child make small sentences? _____

At what age did your child use more complete sentences? _____

Has your child talked better than he or she does now? _____

Does your child appear to be aware of his or her speech differences? _____

What is your child's reaction to his or her speech? _____

Is your child teased about his or her speech by others? _____

When and by whom were your child's speech differences first noticed? _____

What efforts have been made to help your child talk better? _____

Did anyone talk baby-talk to the child? _____ If so, whom? _____

Were your child's wants usually anticipated before he or she could communicate the needs? _____

Did your child gesture much in attempting to communicate? _____

Do you think the child's present vocabulary is superior, average, or inferior to that of other children the same age? _____

Would you consider the child very talkative, average, or rather silent and quiet? _____

Was any foreign language taught to the child or commonly spoken by associates? _____

How well is the child understood?   By parents _____

                                    By peers _____

SCHOOL

Rate your child's school experience related to *academic learning:*

	Good	**Average**	**Poor**
Nursery school	_____	_____	_____
Kindergarten	_____	_____	_____
Current grade	_____	_____	_____

To the best of your knowledge, at what grade level is your child functioning:

Reading _____ Spelling _____ Math _____

Has your child repeated a grade? _____ If so, when? _____

Present class placement _____ Regular class? _____

Kinds of therapy or remedial work your child is receiving _____

Describe any academic school problems _____

Does your child's teacher describe any of the following as significant problems?

Does not sit still in seat	_____
Gets up and walks around room	_____
Shouts out; does not want to be called on	_____
Won't wait his or her turn	_____
Does not cooperate well in groups	_____
Does better one to one	_____
Does not respect other's rights	_____
Does not pay attention	_____

Describe briefly any other classroom problems _____

Peer Relationships:

Does your child seek friends his or her own age? _____

Does your child play primarily with children his or her own age? _____

Younger _____ Older _____

Describe briefly problems the child may have with peers _____

HOME BEHAVIORS

All children exhibit, to some degree, the kinds of behavior listed below. Check those that you believe your child exhibits to an excessive or exaggerated degree when compared with other children of similar age.

Hyperactivity (high activity level)   _____

Poor attention span   _____

Impulsivity (poor self-control)   _____

Low frustration threshold   _____

Temper outbursts   _____

Sloppy table manners   _____

Interrupts frequently   _____

Does not listen when spoken to   _____

Sudden outburst of physical abuse to others   _____

Acts like he or she is driven by a motor   _____

Wears out shoes more frequently than siblings   _____

Pays no attention to danger   _____

Too many accidents   _____

Does not learn from experience   _____

Poor memory   _____

More active than siblings   _____

INTERESTS AND ACCOMPLISHMENTS

What is the child's main interest? _____

What are your child's greatest accomplishments? _____

What does your child enjoy doing most? _____

What does your child dislike doing most? _____

MEDICAL HISTORY

If your child's medical history includes any of the following, please note the age when the accident or illness occurred and any other pertinent information.

Childhood diseases (describe complications) _____

_____

Operations _____

Hospitalizations (other than operations) _____

Head injuries _____

    With unconsciousness _____ Without unconsciousness _____

Convulsions _____ With fever _____ Without fever _____

Coma _____

Meningitis or encephalitis _____

Persistent high fevers _____ Highest temperature recorded _____

Ear problems _____ Eye problems _____

Poisoning _____

Child's physician _____
                         (name, address, telephone number)

PRESENT MEDICAL STATUS

Present height _____ Weight _____

Present illness for which child is being treated _____

Medications taken on an ongoing basis _____

FAMILY HISTORY: *Mother*

Age _____ Age at time of pregnancy with this child _____

Number of previous miscarriages _____

Number of induced abortions _____

School: Highest grade completed _____

        Problems in school _____

Medical problems (specify) _____

Family history of problems similar to child's _____

FAMILY HISTORY: *Father*

Age _____ Age at time of this child's conception _____

School: Highest grade completed _____

        Problems in school _____

Medical problems (specify) _____

Family history of problems similar to child's _____

SIBLINGS: *Name*   *Age*   *Medical — Social — School Problems*

1. _____

2. _____

3. _____

4. _____

5. _____

LIST NAMES AND ADDRESSES OF ANY OTHER PROFESSIONALS CONSULTED

1. _____

2. _____

3. _____

4. _____

Please describe your expectations and hopes for your child as a result of the services you will receive through this agency.

_____

_____

_____

_____

_____

SAMPLE 2

CHILD'S HISTORY FORM

Instructions to parents: Please complete this form to the best of your knowledge and return it. If a question is not applicable to your child, place an N/A in the space provided. If you need more space to answer a particular question, you may attach a separate sheet.

Child's name _____ Sex _____ Birth date _____

Home address _____

_____ Zip _____

Home telephone number _____

Mother's name _____ Father's name _____

Mother's employer _____ Telephone _____

Address _____ Zip _____

Father's employer _____ Telephone _____

Address _____ Zip _____

Pediatrician _____ Telephone _____

Address _____

_____ Zip _____

Insurance company _____ ID # _____

Name of person completing this form _____

Relationship to child _____

Date _____

I. FAMILY HISTORY

Father's age _____ Present occupation _____

Education (highest level) _____

Did father have any developmental delays, speech problems, or special learning problems? _____ If yes, please describe _____

_____

Mother's age _____ Present occupation _____

Education (highest level) _____

Did mother have any developmental delays, speech problems, or special learning problems? _____ If yes, please describe _____

_____

Children:

Name	Age	Any Problems
_____	_____	_____
_____	_____	_____
_____	_____	_____
_____	_____	_____

Other person living in the home:

Name	Age	Relation to Child
_____	_____	_____
_____	_____	_____
_____	_____	_____

Did anyone in the immediate family or any relatives have any of the following? If so, who?

	Yes	No	Who
Neurologic disease	_____	_____	_____
Seizures (epilepsy)	_____	_____	_____
Hearing problems	_____	_____	_____
Visual problems	_____	_____	_____
Emotional problems	_____	_____	_____
Mental retardation	_____	_____	_____
Hyperactivity	_____	_____	_____
Learning problems	_____	_____	_____
Similar problems to the child	_____	_____	_____
Does any disease run in the family?	_____	_____	_____

II. BIRTH HISTORY

Was the child adopted? _____ If so, at what age? _____ Date _____

Did the father or mother have a history of infertility? _____

When was the mother first aware of the pregnancy? (How soon after conception?) _____

In what month of pregnancy did the mother first visit the physician? _____

Were there any miscarriages before this pregnancy? _____

Did the mother have any of the following complications during this pregnancy? Check those that apply.

Anemia	_____	High blood pressure	_____
Swollen ankles	_____	Kidney disease	_____
Heart disease	_____	X-ray exposure	_____
German measles	_____	Toxemia	_____
Staining	_____	Bleeding	_____
Vomiting	_____	Virus	_____
Emotional stress	_____	Nutritional problems	_____
Early labor	_____	Rh incompatability	_____
Accident or injury	_____	Other	_____

Describe _____

_____

_____

Chronic illnesses during pregnancy _____

_____

Did the mother smoke or drink alcoholic beverages during this pregnancy? If so, how much? _____

Did the mother take any medications during this pregnancy? If so, what? _____

Where was the child born?   Home _____   Hospital _____

Name of physician who delivered child _____

Address _____ Telephone _____

How many hours from first contraction to birth? _____

Was the baby early? _____ Late _____

Was the mother given medications during labor? _____

If so, what? _____ Why? _____

Was the mother under anesthesia during childbirth? _____

If so, what kind? _____

Was labor induced? _____ Why? _____

Was the baby born head first? _____

Were forceps used? _____

Did the mother have a cesarean section? _____ Why? _____

Did the baby have any bruises? _____

Did the baby have any birthmarks? _____

Was this a multiple birth? _____

Did the baby have any breathing problems? _____

Was the cord wrapped around the neck? _____

Did the baby cry quickly? _____

Was the baby's color normal? _____ Describe _____

What was the baby's Apgar score at 1 minute? _____ 5 minutes? _____

If the baby was jaundiced (yellow), did he or she receive:

    Oxygen   Yes _____   No _____   How long? _____

    Transfusions   Yes _____   No _____   How long? _____

    Phototherapy   Yes _____   No _____   How long? _____

Birth weight: _____ lbs. _____ oz.

Were there any physical defects? _____

Any complications before the baby went home? _____

Was the baby placed in an incubator or special crib? _____ How long? _____

How long after birth did the baby go home? _____

III. DEVELOPMENTAL HISTORY

A. General

Was the baby breast-fed? _____ Bottle-fed? _____

Did the baby have feeding problems? _____ Describe _____

Was the baby colicky? _____ How long? _____

Did the baby require formula changes? _____

Difficulty sucking as an infant? _____ Describe _____

Was the baby normally active? Yes _____ No _____ Describe _____

Was the baby limp? _____ Describe _____

Was the baby stiff? _____ Describe _____

Did the baby show any unusual trembling? _____

Did the baby fail to grow normally? _____

Did the baby fail to gain weight? _____

Was the baby different in any way from siblings? _____

B. Motor development

How old was the child when he or she:

Sat alone _____ Stood alone _____ Crawled _____

Walked alone _____ Fed self _____ Toilet trained _____

Was the baby's motor development average? _____ Fast _____ Slow _____

C. Speech/language development

How old was the baby when he or she:

Babbled and cooed _____ Noticed others talking _____

Spoke first words _____ Combined two or three words _____

Spoke first sentences _____

Was the child's speech development average? _____ Fast _____ Slow _____

IV. MEDICAL/HEALTH INFORMATION

Has the child ever had:

Yes		Age	Severity	Change in Development
_____	Encephalitis	_____	_____	_____
_____	Meningitis	_____	_____	_____
_____	Fever of 104°F	_____	_____	_____
_____	Allergies	_____	_____	_____
_____	Asthma	_____	_____	_____
_____	Draining ears	_____	_____	_____
_____	Ear infections	_____	_____	_____
_____	Convulsions or seizures	_____	_____	_____

Describe any other serious illnesses _____

_____

Describe any loss of consciousness _____

_____

Describe any surgeries _____

_____

Is the child currently taking any medications? _____ Describe _____

_____

Are there any restrictions on the child's activities? _____
   Describe _____

Have you consulted any medical specialists for the child? _____
   If so, who? _____ When _____
   Results _____

Indicate the date of the last physical examination _____
   Physician _____

Indicate the child's present health _____

Indicate any special recommendations by the physician _____

V. BEHAVIOR AND SOCIAL HISTORY

Please indicate which of these traits are characteristic:

Is the child:

_____	Nervous	_____	Destructive
_____	Well-behaved	_____	Easily discouraged
_____	Clumsy	_____	Easily excitable
_____	Impulsive	_____	Selfish
_____	Stubborn	_____	Jealous
_____	Shy	_____	Poor eater
_____	Showoff	_____	Picky eater
_____	Rude	_____	Slow to respond
_____	Distractable	_____	Quick to respond

Does the child:

_____	Wet bed	_____	Set fires
_____	Have nightmares	_____	Suck thumb
_____	Walk in sleep	_____	Have temper tantrums
_____	Refuse to obey	_____	Steal
_____	Run away when called	_____	Lie
_____	Whine frequently	_____	Fight with others
_____	Hurt pets	_____	Prefer older children
_____	Drool	_____	Prefer younger children
_____	Hit, kick, hurt others	_____	Eat inedible objects
_____	Bang the head	_____	Have blank spells
_____	Repeat activities for prolonged periods	_____	Have toilet accidents during the day

How long will the child pay attention to preferred activities (television, games)?
_____

How well does the child interact with adults? _____

How well does the child interact with other children? _____

Has the child had any unusual or traumatic experiences? _____
  Describe _____

Does the child have any unusual fears? _____
  Describe _____

Are there significant marital conflicts in the home? _____

Are there significant conflicts between the child and the parents? _____
  Describe _____

Are there significant conflicts between the children? _____

Do the parents agree on how to discipline the child? _____

What types of discipline are most effective? _____

Does the child demand attention from the parents? _____

How does the child relate to the mother? _____ Father _____

What do you enjoy doing with the child? _____

What types of play does the child enjoy most? _____

What are the child's favorite toys? _____

Describe what the child does on a typical day _____
_____

What are the child's favorite foods? _____

What time does the child go to bed? _____ Awaken? _____

VI. MISCELLANEOUS

Which hand does the child prefer? _____

Are there languages other than English spoken in the home? _____

How well does the family understand the child's speech? _____

Describe the child's movements: Sluggish _____ Active _____ Constant _____

VII. CONCERN AND PREVIOUS EVALUATIONS

Who was the first to express concern about the child? _____
  When? _____ Why? _____

Has any change taken place since that time? _____
  Describe _____

To what do you attribute that change? _____

Has the child had emotional, adjustment, or behavioral problems? _____
  Describe _____

Has the child received any psychiatric or psychological treatment? _____
  Describe _____

Do you suspect a hearing problem? _____ Vision problem? _____

Have any of the following been used by other professionals to describe the child?

  _____ Autistic   _____ Brain damaged

  _____ Cerebral palsied   _____ Mentally retarded

  _____ Gifted   _____ Developmentally delayed

  _____ Other   Describe _____

VIII. DAY CARE AND SCHOOL HISTORY

Day care or school now attending _____

Teacher name _____ School telephone _____

Does the child like school? _____ Like teacher? _____

Is child frequently absent? _____ Describe _____

Any problems with the day care or school? _____

What feedback have you received about the child's school performance? _____

Is there anything else about the child that you feel we should know? If so, please describe in detail below.

SAMPLE 3

HIGH-RISK FOLLOW-UP CLINIC PROGRAM

Name _____ Parent's name _____

Date of birth _____ Address _____

_____ Telephone _____

Visit # _____ Number of siblings _____

Date _____ Chronologic age _____

Primary care physician _____

SUMMARY OF RISK FACTORS

BW _____ Gestation _____ AGA _____ SGA _____ LGA _____

RDS _____ BPD _____ Prolonged ventilation _____

Chest tube _____ Apgars _____ , _____

Asphyxia _____ IVH _____ RLF _____

Neurodevelopmental examination results at discharge _____

_____

Other anomalies _____

Other risk factors _____

Other issues _____

HISTORY OF PRESENT ILLNESS

Parental concerns _____

_____

_____

Recent illnesses _____

Apnea monitor _____ Problems _____

INTERIM HISTORY

Nutrition _____

    Problems _____

Elimination problems _____

Sleep patterns _____

Surgeries _____

Immunizations _____

Medications _____

DEVELOPMENTAL HISTORY AND CARETAKERS

Clinical, linguistic, and auditory milestones (CLAMS) _____
_____
_____
_____

Visual and fine motor milestones _____
_____
_____

Family history _____

    Parents _____

    Caretakers _____

    Problems and care issues _____
_____

    Other issues (family) _____
_____

PHYSICAL EXAMINATION

Weight _____ Percentile _____ Length _____ Percentile _____

General _____
_____

HEENT _____

Lungs _____

CV _____

Abdomen _____

Genitalia _____

Extremities _____

NEURODEVELOPMENTAL EXAMINATION

Cranial nerves _____
_____

Vision _____ _____
_____

Auditory _____

Muscle tone _____

Primitive reflex profile: Positive support _____ DRBB _____ ATNR _____

Galant _____ STL _____ PTL _____ STNR _____ MORO _____

Asymmetries _____ Pathologic reflexes _____

Deep tendon reflexes _____

Postural responses _____

Highest motor achievement _____

Coordination, involuntary movements _____

Asymmetries _____

Visual, problem-solving skills _____

Clinical, linguistic, auditory examination _____

BEHAVIORAL OBSERVATIONS

Attention _____

Interaction _____

Behaviors _____

BAYLEY ASSESSMENT

SPECIAL STUDIES

IMPRESSION

_____
_____
_____
_____
_____
_____

DIAGNOSES

_____
_____
_____
_____
_____
_____

PLAN

_____
_____
_____
_____
_____
_____

INFANT STIMULATION PROGRAM GOALS

Language _____
_____
_____

Social and adaptive _____
_____
_____

Problem solving _____
_____
_____

Gross and fine motor _____
_____
_____

SERVICES TO RECEIVE COPIES

_____
_____

APPENDIX B

*Annotated Bibliography
of Infant and Child
Assessment Instruments*

The material contained in this appendix was adapted, in part, from publications obtained from the Minnesota Department of Education and the Illinois Department of Specialized Educational Services. The specific publications are listed below:

Bettenburg, A. (1985). *Instruments and procedures for assessing young children.* St. Paul: Minnesota Department of Education.

Smith, S., and Rudnall, R. (1982). *Early childhood assessment: Recommended practices and selected instruments.* Springfield: Illinois State Board of Education.

Test Name: *Assessing Prelinguistic and Early Linguistic Behaviors in Developmentally Young Children* (1987)

Authors: L. Olswang, C. Stoel-Gammons, T. Coggins, and R. Carpenter.

Publisher: University of Washington Press, Seattle, WA   98145

Purpose/Description: *Assessing Prelinguistic and Early Linguistic Behaviors* is a manual describing an assessment protocol for children functioning between 9 and 24 months of age. The program includes five scales assessing the following aspects of prelinguistic and early linguistic development: cognitive antecedents to word meaning; play; communicative intent; language comprehension; and language production.

Test Name: *Assessment in Infancy: Ordinal Scales of Psychological Development* (1975)

Author(s): I. C. Uzgiris and J. Hunt

Publisher: University of Illinois Press

Address: Box 5081, Station A, Champaign, IL   61820

Purpose/Description: The six ordinal scales measure the effects of infants' encounters with various kinds of circumstances in relation to cognitive development. This assessment tool uses Piaget's work and is based on the theory that development is a process of evolving new, more complex, hierarchical levels of organization, intellect, and motivation. Six individually administered scales have been developed to measure infant development. It is not necessary to present the scales in a single session or in sequence, nor is it necessary to administer all the scales. It is necessary, however, to present situations appropriate for eliciting the critical actions for several consecutive steps on the scale to ascertain the infant's level of development. The populations examined in developing the scales ranged in age from 1 to 24 months.

Test Name: *Attachment-Separation-Individuation Scale* (ASI) (1981)

Author(s): B. Mosey

Publisher: The Family Centered Resource Project — Outreach
Address: 3010 St. Lawrence Avenue, Reading, PA 19602 (215) 779-7111

Purpose/Description: The purpose of the ASI is to provide informal evaluation of the social and emotional interactions between infant and parents. The evaluator assesses three parameters: (1) the infant's attachment–separation–individuation-oriented behaviors, (2) parent behaviors in relation to encouragement and discouragement of the child's behaviors, and (3) the parent-child interaction. No quantifiable score is obtained, but a rating score is developed to identify where parent and child are on the continuum of attachment-separation-individuation development. Administration takes up to one hour depending on the child's age. The scale is designed for subjects ranging from infancy to 3 years.

Test: *Battelle Developmental Inventory* (BDI) (1984)
Author(s): J. Newborg, J. Stock, and L. Wnek
Publisher: DLM Teaching Resources
Address: One DLM Park, Allen, TX 75002

Purpose/Description: One of the primary functions of the BDI is to identify children who are handicapped or delayed in several areas of development. The BDI includes a screening test that can be used to identify those areas of development in which a child needs comprehensive assessment with the complete BDI. The BDI is a standardized, individually administered assessment battery of key developmental skills. It consists of a screening component and a full battery. The full BDI consists of 341 test items grouped into five domains: personal-social, adaptive, motor, communication, and cognitive. Each domain is contained in a separate test booklet. The BDI screening test consists of 96 of the 341 items. Each item is presented in a standard format that specifies the behavior to be assessed, the materials needed for testing, the procedures for administering the item, and the criteria for scoring. Data are collected through presentation of a structured test format, interviews with parents and teachers, and observations of the child in a natural setting. The instrument can be administered to children ranging in age from birth to 8 years. Modifications are suggested for children with motor, visual, and auditory impairments.

Test: *Bayley Scales of Infant Development* (1969)
Author(s): N. Bayley
Publisher: Psychological Corporation
Address: 304 East 45th Street, New York, NY 10017

Purpose/Description: The Bayley scales assess developmental status in infants and young children. The instrument consists of two scales. The mental scale (163 items) measures (1) sensory-perceptual acuities and discrimination; (2) early acquisition of object constancy and memory, learning, and problem-solving ability; (3) vocalizations and the beginning of verbal communication; and (4) early evidence of the ability to form generalizations and classifications. The motor scale (81 items) measures the degree and control of body coordination of the large muscles and finer manipulatory skills of the hands and fingers. The infant behavior record, which consists of 30 ratings, is completed after the scales have been administered and on the basis of the examiner's observation. The scales can be administered to children aged 2 to 30 months.

Test Name: *Birth to Three Assessment and Intervention System*
Author(s): T. Bangs
Publisher: DLM Teaching Resources
Address: One DLM Park, Allen, TX 75002

Purpose/Description: The *Birth to Three Assessment and Intervention System* consists of three parts: the screening test of learning and language development, the checklist of learning and language behavior, and the intervention manual. It is designed to identify, measure, and address developmental delays in children aged 0 to 3 years. The system provides both a norm-referenced screening test and a criterion-referenced checklist of skills. The scores obtained may be computed into standard scores, percentile ranks, and stanines. The system includes items covering language comprehension, language expression, problem solving, social-personal skills, and motor development.

Test Name: *Bracken Basic Concept Scale* (BBCS) (1984)
Author(s): B. A. Bracken
Publisher: Charles E. Merrill
Address: Bell & Howell Company, Columbus, OH 43216

Purpose/Description: The BBCS allows for an in-depth assessment of an individual child's conceptual knowledge. A screening version of the scale is also available to identify which children may benefit from a more intensive diagnostic assessment. The BBCS measures 258 concepts divided into 11 categories or subtests: colors, letter identification, numbers-counting, comparisons, shapes, direction-position, social-emotional, size, texture-material, quantity, and time-sequence. The BBCS yields the following scores: (1) the first five listed subtests are combined for a school readiness composite standard score, (2) the remaining six subtests have individual scores, and (3) a composite score that is a total of the standard scores for the 11 subtests. A 30-item screening test is also available, which is intended to be used primarily with kindergarten and first-grade children. The test format requires that the examiner read a statement and the child respond by pointing. No verbal responses are required. The diagnostic scale of the BBCS is appropriate for children between 2 years, 6 months, and 7 years, 11 months. The BBCS screening test is appropriate for children aged 5 to 7 years.

Test Name: *California Preschool Social Competency Scale*
Author(s): S. Levine, F. F. Elzey, and M. Lewis
Publisher: Consulting Psychological Press, Inc.
Address: 577 College Avenue, Palo Alto, CA 94306

Purpose/Description: This scale is designed to measure the adequacy of interpersonal behavior and degree of social responsibility in children ages 2 to 5 years. The behaviors included are situational. They were selected in terms of common cultural expectations to represent basic competencies to be developed in the process of socialization. The scale contains 30 items. Each item consists of four descriptive statements, given in behavioral terms, and represents various degrees of competency. The examiner must have had considerable opportunity to observe the child in a variety of situations prior to completing the scale. The scale was designed for use with children ranging in age from 2½ to 5½ years.

Test Name: *Carolina Developmental Profile* (CDP) (1975)
Author(s): D. L. Lillie and G. L. Harbin
Publisher: Kaplan School Supply Corporation
Address: 600 Jonestown Road, Winston-Salem, NC 27103

Purpose/Description: The CDP is an individually administered criterion-referenced test consisting of a test booklet with instructions included on the inside cover and a profile on the back cover. The CDP covers developmental abilities in six areas: gross motor, fine motor, visual perception, reasoning, receptive language, and expressive language. It is designed to be used with the developmental task instruction system. In this system, the goal is to increase the child's developmental abilities to the maximum level of proficiency to prepare the child for the formal academic tasks that will be faced in the early elementary school years. The profile is designed to assist the teacher in establishing long-range objectives to increase developmental abilities in six areas. The purpose of the checklist is not to compare or assess the child in terms of age-normative data. The CDP can be used with children from 2 to 5 years.

Test Name: *Cognitive Observation Guide* (COG)
Author(s): B. Mosey
Publisher: The Family Centered Research Project — Outreach
Address: 3010 St. Lawrence Avenue, Reading, PA 19606 (215) 779-7711

Purpose/Description: The COG is designed to provide a conceptual and behavioral framework for assessing and facilitating cognitive skills in young children. An informal criterion-referenced observation guide for assessing cognition, the COG is composed of 24 subskills with behavioral indicators arranged by age level. Each item or behavioral indicator is scored individually. Results are informal and indicate the child's progress toward developing specific cognitive skills. It is designed for use with subjects from birth to 2 years.

Test Name: *Denver Developmental Screening Test* (DDST) (1968, 1970, 1973)
Author(s): W. K. Frankenburg, J. B. Dodds, and A. W. Fandal
Publisher: William K. Frankenburg and Josiah B. Dodds
Address: Lacoda Project and Publishing Foundation, Inc., East 51st Avenue and Lincoln Street, Denver, CO 80216

Purpose/Description: The DDST was designed and standardized as a simple, useful tool to aid in the early discovery of children with developmental problems. A screening instrument, it is not intended to diagnose specific problems. The DDST is an individually administered screening test of development with 105 items arranged in four sectors: personal-social, fine motor–adaptive, language, and gross motor. The test can be administered to children from 2 weeks to 6 years.

Test Name: *Developmental Activities Screening Inventory* (DASI) (1977)
Author(s): R. F. DuBose and M. B. Langley
Publisher: Teaching Resources
Address: 50 Pond Park Road, Hingham, MD 02808

Purpose/Description: The main purpose of the authors was to design an easily administered screening test that could be used with preschool handicapped children. The test has a nonverbal design so that children with auditory impairments or language disorders would not be penalized by their handicap. The test has modifications for the visually impaired. The DASI kit is equipped with a carrying case, an instructor guide, and educational materials for administering the test. Everyday objects, necessary for administration, are not included; scoring sheets are. The DASI is an informal, individually administered test. The tasks are presented to the child through demonstration, and the child's response is observed and recorded on a checklist score sheet. Areas that are measured include fine motor coordination, cause-effect and means-end relationship, association, number concepts, size discrimination, and seriation. The DASI is designed as an informal screening measure for children functioning between the ages of 6 and 60 months.

Test Name: *Developmental Indicators for Assessment of Learning* (rev.) (DIAL-R) (1983)
Author(s): C. D. Mardell-Czudnowski and D. Goldenberg
Publisher: Childcraft Education Corporation
Address: 20 Kilmer Road, Edison, NJ 08818

Purpose/Description: DIAL-R is an early childhood screening test that is intended to assist in the identification of children who may have special education needs. The DIAL-R can be used to determine if further assessment or diagnosis of a child must be completed in accordance with state and federal mandates for serving young handicapped children. The authors also indicate that the DIAL-R can be used in the regular classroom to identify students' strengths and weaknesses as the first step in programming or curriculum development. The DIAL-R was revised in 1983 and is considered to be an improved version of the original DIAL screening instrument. It is a team-administered individual assessment of early childhood development. The basic format and procedures of the original DIAL are maintained on the DIAL-R, and it assesses the following areas: motor, concepts, and language. The norms have also been extended to include children from 2 to 6 years of age. It includes separate norms for white and nonwhite populations.

Test Name: *The Developmental Profile*
Author(s): G. Alpern and T. Boll
Publisher: Psychological Development Corporation
Address: P.O. Box 3198, Aspen, CO 81611

Purpose/Description: *The Developmental Profile* is an inventory of skills that has been designed to assess a child's development from birth to preadolescence. *The Developmental Profile* consists of 217 items arranged into five scales. All scales have the items arranged into age levels. The age levels proceed in six-month intervals from birth to 3½ years and proceed thereafter by year intervals. Year intervals describe children 6 months from both sides of the year norms (e.g., 6-year level covers ages 5½ to 6½ years). The profile is administered in an interview format with a rater who knows the child well. The rater might also self-administer the test. The scale can be used with children ranging from birth to 12 years. The authors indicate that the scale can be used for assessing handicapped children. However, some revisions must be made with test administration procedures.

Test Name: *Diagnostic Inventory of Early Development* (Brigance) (1978)
Author(s): A. H. Brigance
Publisher: Curriculum Associates
Address: 5 Esquire Road North, Billerica, MA 01862 (800) 225-0246

Purpose/Description: The Brigance inventory was designed to simplify and combine the processes of assessing, diagnosing, recordkeeping, and instructional planning for young children. The author claims that the instrument serves as an assessment instrument, an instructional guide, a recordkeeping tracking system, and tool for developing and communicating an individualized education plan (IEP), and a resource for training parents and professionals. The individually administered inventory includes 98 skill sequences, from birth through the developmental age of 6 years, for the following areas: psychomotor, self-help, speech and language, general knowledge and comprehension, and early academic skills. It is criterion referenced but is considered by the author to be norm referenced because the age ranges for each skill were validated from several resources that list normative data. During administration the inventory booklet is opened to an assessment procedure, and the printed material for the examiner is in the correct position for reading with the visual materials facing the child. The author recommends that the materials provided by the examiner to assess the child be familiar to the child and commonly found in the home or school. The inventory was designed to be used in programs for infants and children below the developmental age of 7 years.

Test Name: *Diagnostic Inventory for Screening Children* (DISC)
Author(s): J. Amdur, M. Mainland, and K. Parker
Publisher: The Psychological Corporation
Address: San Antonio, TX 78283

Purpose/Description: The DISC is a diagnostic screening instrument for use with children from birth through 5 years of age. The DISC determines average–above average functioning or possible–probable delay in eight developmental areas. The instrument takes 15 to 40 minutes to administer. Percentile equivalents or raw scores are provided for the eight scales for each of 11 age groups. Interpretive tables based on the percentiles are available for each of the eight scales. The eight domains assessed are fine motor skills, gross motor skills, and receptive language; expressive language; visual attention and memory; auditory attention and memory; self-help skills; and social skills. Examiner training exercises are available in a videotape format.

Test Name: *The Early Intervention Developmental Profile* (Developmental Programming for Infants and Young Children) (Vols. 1–3, 1977; Vols. 4 and 5, 1981)
Author(s): D. S. Schafer and M. S. Moersch
Publisher: The University of Michigan Press
Address: 615 East University, Ann Arbor, MI 48106

Purpose/Description: Volumes 1, 2, 4, and 5 enable the educator or therapist to develop comprehensive and individualized developmental programs by translating comprehensive evaluation data rendered by the profile into short-term behavioral objectives that form the basis of daily living activities planned to facilitate emerging skills. Volume 3, a comprehensive collection of sequenced activities, enables parents and professionals to select appropriate activities that will blend into the family's daily routine (birth to 36 months). *Assessment and Application,* Volumes 1 and 4, and *The Early Intervention Developmental Profile,* make up the assessment portion of the program. This assessment instrument is made up of six scales that provide developmental milestones in the following areas: perceptual–fine motor, cognition, language, social-emotional, self-care, and gross motor development. The profile contains 487 items and yields information for planning comprehensive developmental programs for children with various handicaps who function below the 72-month level. The five-volume program has been designed for children aged birth to 72 months.

Test Name: *Environmental Language Inventory* (ELI)
Author(s): J. D. MacDonald and M. Nichols
Publisher: Charles E. Merrill
Address: 1300 Alum Creek Drive, Columbus, OH 43216

Purpose/Description: The instrument offers both a diagnostic and training design for clinical work with children demonstrating severe delay in expressive language. The ELI consists of procedures to assess expressive language in three modes: imitation, conversation, and play. Imitation and conversation may be assessed in a single procedure. A separate procedure is provided for assessing expressive language in free play. Test materials include the manual and recording forms. The examiner must gather additional materials. The following scores are available from the ELI: frequency, rank order, and proportion of semantic-grammatical rules, utterance length, proportion of intelligible words; and frequency of unintelligible words. These scores are provided for each of the three modes. The ELI is appropriately used for children whose communication is primarily limited to one- and two-word utterances with minimal spontaneous production. The ELI assesses expressive language from the first word combinations through four-word sentences.

Test Name: *Environmental Pre-Language Battery* (EPB)
Author(s): D. S. Horstmeier and J. D. MacDonald
Publisher: Charles E. Merrill
Address: 1300 Alum Creek Drive, Columbus, OH 43216

Purpose/Description: The EPB can be used primarily for two purposes: for diagnostic assessment of individual children before prescriptive training and for prelanguage and postlanguage program evaluation using the scores shown on the summary sheet. Each child's growth can be shown in a percentage of change. Training packets keyed to the EPB diagnostic levels are available in a language training manual designed to be used by parents, language therapists, teachers, and other concerned individuals. Seven prelanguage and early language levels are covered in the EPB diagnostic assessment: (1) preliminary skills, (2) functional play with objects, (3) motor imitation, (4) receptive language, (5) sound imitation, (6) single word imitation, and (7) beginning social conversation. The battery is intended for use with language-delayed children functioning below or at the single-word level.

Test Name: *Flint Infant Security Scale* (1974)
Author(s): B. M. Flint
Publisher: Guidance Center
Address: Faculty of Education, University of Toronto, Toronto, Canada M4W 2K8

Purpose/Description: The Flint security scale is designed to assess the mental and emotional health of children from 3 months to 2 years of age. Applications to pediatric examinations, preadoptive placements, and implications for intervention therapies are provided. The scale has a total of 72 items describing infant-toddler behavior. These items describe a range of behavior and encompass a variety of life experiences. Through an interview with the mother and objective descriptions of the child's observed behavior while in the same room during the interview, security ratings or scores are obtained in the following eight areas: eating, unfamiliar situation, sleeping, toileting and bathing, physical experience, changing environment, socializing, and playing. The rating choices are "secure" versus "deputing agent and regression." The former is a positive, healthy, and age-appropriate rating, and the latter is a negative, unhealthy, and age-inappropriate rating.

Test Name: *Functional Profile* (1981)
Author(s): Peoria 0-3 Program, Allied Agencies Center
Publisher: Materials Coordinator, The Peoria 0-3 Outreach Project

Address: 320 East Armstrong Avenue, Peoria, IL 61603

Purpose/Description: The *Functional Profile* is designed to determine an approximate level of functioning and to plan a program suited to the child's individual needs. The profile is a checklist of 481 developmental skills and social traits that normal infants and young children usually demonstrate at certain age levels. There are seven categories: social, cognitive-linguistic-verbal, gross motor, fine motor, eating, dressing, and toileting. Within each category the tasks are separated into age groups in months and are arranged according to level of difficulty. The levels and ceilings are established in the usual manner. The child's performance is rated either "yes" or "no," the behavior being present or absent. The child is said to be functioning at the highest level at which one more than half the items are passed. Functioning levels are plotted on a graph to provide a visual representation of the child's skills. The profile is designed for use with children ranging in age from birth to 6 years.

Test Name: *Gesell Developmental Schedules* (1940)
Author(s): A. Gesell
Publisher: Nigel Cox
Address: 69 Fawn Drive, Cheshire, CT 06410

Purpose/Description: The *Gesell Developmental Schedules* were developed and organized to provide an adequate developmental diagnosis. The diagnosis requires an examination of the quality and integration of five domains of behavior. The *Gesell Developmental Schedules* are individually administered and assess five domains of behavior: adaptive, gross motor, fine motor, language, and personal-social. The materials required for the developmental examination are contained in a kit, but no manual is provided. The user will need to refer to *Developmental Diagnoses* (Knobloch and Pasamanick, 1974) for a discussion of the schedules and assessment procedures. The schedules are designed for children aged 4 weeks to 6 years.

Test Name: *Griffiths Mental Development Scales* (1954)
Author(s): R. Griffiths
Publisher: Test Center, Inc.
Address: Snug Harbor Village, 7221 Holiday Drive, Sarasota, FL 33581

Purpose/Description: The Griffiths scales were designed to measure trends of development that indicate mental growth in young children (standardized measure of intelligence). They are divided into two levels: birth to 2 years, which is described in *The Abilities of Babies,* and 2 to 8 years, which is described in *The Abilities of Young Children.* Five scales are used in evaluating the birth to 2-year-old child: locomotion, personal-social, hearing and speech, eye and hand coordination, and performance. A sixth scale, practical reasoning, is added for children 3 to 8 years. A developmental age and developmental quotient can be computed for each scale as well as an overall mental age and intelligence quotient.

Test: *Hawaii Early Learning Profile* (HELP) (1979)
Author(s): Enrichment Project for Handicapped Infants (S. Furuno, Director)
Publisher: VORT Corporation
Address: P.O. Box 11132, Palo Alto, CA 94306

Purpose/Description: The HELP was developed to assist in planning individualized programs for children with a wide range of handicaps and diagnoses. It provides a comprehensive visual picture of the child's functioning levels and focuses on the whole child (i.e., building strengths as well as helping work on areas of weakness). The HELP is divided into the HELP charts and the HELP activity guide. The chart provides a comprehensive visual picture, and the skills are developmentally sequenced in small incremental steps, arranged in a horizontal continuum. The guide corresponds with the developmental steps and assists in planning and task analysis to develop the appropriate skills. Both the chart and guide provide a month-to-month sequence of normal developmental skills in six areas: cognitive, expressive language, gross motor, fine motor, self-help, and social-emotional. The profile is intended for use with children from birth to 36 months.

Test: *Home Observation for Measurement of the Environment* (HOME) (1978)
Author(s): B. M. Caldwell
Publisher: Child Development Research Unit
Address: University of Arkansas at Little Rock, 33rd and University Avenue, Little Rock, AR 72204

Purpose/Description: Two separate instruments have been designed to sample certain aspects of the quantity and quality of social, emotional, and cognitive support available to a young child within the child's home. Only one instrument measures these aspects for children from birth to age 3 years. The second measures these aspects for children from ages 3 to 6. The inventory for children ages birth to 3 contains 45 items; the inventory for 3- to 6-year-old children contains 55 items. The original intent was that all items would be based on direct observation of the interaction between caretaker (usually the mother) and the child. However, an examination of the item pool suggested that many important areas of experience for the infant and preschooler were excluded with this restriction on item selection. Therefore, succeeding versions of the inventory included items requiring an interview format. Such items make up about one third of the total number for the birth to 3-years inventory and about two-thirds of the total number for the 3- to 6-years inventory. The present version of each of the inventories requires a home visit of about one hour when the child is awake. The instructional manuals provide a description of items, definitions, guidelines for conducting the interviews, and recommendations for reducing subjectivity on scoring. The inventory for infants can be used for children from birth to 3 years of age. The preschool version is intended for children aged 3 to 6 years.

Test Name: *Indiana Preschool Developmental Assessment Scale* (IPDAS) (Indiana Home Teaching System for Parents and Handicapped Pre-schoolers) (1976)
Author(s): Primary authors: B. Bateman, J. Kenn, J. Wilke, R. Wilson, C. Maslen, and W. A. Bragg
Publisher: Developmental Training Center
Address: 2853 East Tenth Street, Bloomington, IN 47401

Purpose/Description: The purpose of the total program (IHTS) is fourfold: (1) to provide a comprehensive model for the home delivery of educational services to handicapped preschool children, (2) to provide an assessment instrument applicable to preschool handicapped children, (3) to develop a corresponding home teaching curriculum and related materials for parental use with the preschool handicapped child, and (4) to provide technical assistance to administrators and professional and paraprofessional service providers at the preschool level. The purpose of this assessment is to develop a well-defined profile describing the level of the child's developmental functioning in the motor, personal autonomy, communication, and preacademic areas. This profile will be used to formulate an appropriate educational program for the child to be carried out generally by the parents under the guidance of a key staff member. The scale is intended for use with children from birth to 6 years.

Test Name: *Infant Intelligence Test* (1940–1960)
Author(s): P. Cattell
Publisher: The Psychological Corporation
Address: 304 East 45th Street, New York, NY 10017

Purpose/Description: As of October 1937, the author was unable to find a single published test for infants that contained definite and precise directions for scoring, comparable to those for children of school age. The infant intelligence scale was constructed to be as free as possible from the limitations of existing infant tests at that time. The scale consists of five items at each month from 2 to 12 months. From 12 to 24 months, five items are presented at two-month intervals. From 24 to 30 months, five items are presented at three-month intervals. Two thirds of the manual is devoted to the administration of test items. Each item is presented on a separate page. The directions include the materials to be used, the procedures to be followed, and the scoring system to be applied. The majority of the items include a photograph that illustrates a young child responding to the task. The materials and examination forms used to administer the test are contained in a small suitcase. The publisher has attempted to organize the case of materials in a manner that facilitates the administration process. The scale's items range developmentally from two to 30 months.

Test Name: *Infant Scale of Communicative Intent*
Author(s): St. Christopher's Hospital for Children
Publisher: St. Christopher's Hospital; *Update Pediatrics,* January 1982, Vol. 7

Purpose/Description: *The Infant Scale of Communicative Intent* is a nonstandardized, descriptive measure developed to meet the needs of a population of infants with developmental problems. The scale was compiled from published tests, research data, and clinical experience. It emphasizes the infant's intent to communicate in several modes and to interact socially with others. The scale consists of a checklist containing ten behaviors at one-month intervals from birth to 18 months of age. The items at each age are intended to provide a general description of the communicative behavior of children at each stage. The scale is administered by observation, direct testing, or parental report.

Test Name: *Koontz Child Developmental Program Training Activities for the First 48 months* (1974)
Author(s): C. W. Koontz
Publisher: Western Psychological Services
Address: 12031 Wilshire Boulevard, Los Angeles, CA 90025

Purpose/Description: The Koontz instrument was designed to evaluate, monitor progress, and plan suitable activities for infants. Evaluation is achieved by matching the behavior of a child in a normal setting with a list of graded observable performance items. Progress is recorded in relation to the performance items, and activities are suggested that are designed to reinforce the performance items. Four functional areas of development are considered: gross motor, fine motor, social, and language. There is a possible total of 550 performance items. Activities associated with each level and each area are designed to strengthen the performance of the items. Other pertinent information corresponding to the levels and the areas is included in the activity section. The program is designed for children aged 1 to 48 months.

Test Name: *Learning Accomplishment Profile: Diagnostic Edition* (LAP-I) (rev.) (1977)
Author(s): D. W. LeMay, P. M. Griffin, and A. R. Sanford
Publisher: Kaplan School Supply Corporation
Address: 600 Jonestown Road, Winston-Salem, NC 27103

Purpose/Description: The LAP-D sees as a major educational objective the determination of the individual child's mastery level in each of the five skill areas included in the instrument. It is anticipated that the accurate and reliable assessment of the child's developmental level should translate into an effective instructional program, providing the foundation in which sound instructional programs can be grounded. The LAP-D consists of 323 items organized according to five scales and 13 subscales: fine motor (manipulating and writing), cognitive (matching and counting), language/cognitive (naming and comprehension), gross motor (body movement and object movement), self-help (eating, dressing, grooming, toileting, and self-direction). The items within each subscale are arranged in ascending order of complexity and in a task-analytic manner. Each item describes the behavior to be observed, the procedure to be followed in eliciting the desired responses, and the criteria against which success is measured. Develomental ages are provided for each item. At six-month intervals the developmental ages serve as indicators of the appropriate starting point for the assessment. The LAP-D kit contains a looseleaf easel that contains the procedures for administering the test, a list of the behaviors to be observed, criteria for evaluating the child's performance, and picture cards and matching cards located in pockets adjacent to the particular items. A variety of colorful materials are also included in the kit. All the materials necessary for complete assessment (except for food items for the self-help section) are provided. Behaviors assessed with the LAP-D range from a developmental age of 6 to 72 months.

Test Name: *Learning Accomplishment Profile for Infants* (Early LAP) (rev.) (1975, rev. 1978)

Author(s): M. E. Glover, J. L. Preminger, and A. R. Sanford
Publisher: Kaplan Press
Address: 600 Jonestown Road, Winston-Salem, NC 27103

Purpose/Description: The Early LAP is a criterion-referenced assessment that provides a simple profile of the overall development of children from birth to 3 years. The Early LAP is a revision of the 1975 *Learning Accomplishment Profile for Infants*. It contains six developmental skill areas: gross motor, fine motor, cognitive, language, self-help, and social-emotional. The 412 items were taken from previously developed instruments. The bibliography lists 19 sources. Items are stated as behavioral objectives. Developmental ages are provided. Individually administered, the instrument is intended for use with children from birth to 36 months.

Test Name: *McCarthy Scales of Children's Abilities* (1972)
Author(s): D. McCarthy
Publisher: The Psychological Corporation
Address: 7955 Caldwell Avenue, Chicago, IL 60648

Purpose/Description: The McCarthy scales were designed to evaluate children's general intellectual level as well as their strengths and weaknesses in a number of ability areas. This individually administered test consists of 18 subtests that make up six scales: verbal, perceptual-performance, quantitative, memory, motor, and general cognitive. The general cognitive scale is a composite of the verbal, perceptual-performance, and quantitative scales. The attractive test materials facilitate the establishment and maintenance of rapport. The sequential organization of the McCarthy scales is an important feature that also promotes the establishment of rapport. The test begins with manipulative items; gross motor tests appear midway when the child is becoming restless and interest is beginning to wane; and the final items require limited vocalizations in anticipation of the child's state of fatigue. The McCarthy scales contain several built-in precautions to promote optimum measurement of the child's ability in each task. Extra trials are permitted for many items to give a child a second chance; only the best performance is counted. To ensure that the child understands the task at hand, he or she is frequently given feedback on the easier items; on one subtest examples are given to get the child started. In addition, the inclusion of several multipoint items rewards the child for virtually any response approximating correct performance. The test can be administered to children from 2½ to 8½ years.

Test Name: *Marshalltown Behavioral Developmental Profile* (copyright pending)
Author(s): M. Donahue, A. F. Keiser, J. C. Montgomery, V. L. Roecker, L. I. Smith, and M. F. Walden
Publisher: The Marshalltown Project
Address: 507 East Anson Street, Marshalltown, IA 50158

Purpose/Description: The purpose is to facilitate individual prescriptive teaching of preschool children within the home setting. There are three developmental categories: communication, motor, and social. A total of 327 items is provided. Each item is briefly stated in behavioral terms; however, no criteria examples are given. A direct test procedure is used; there is no allowance for parent report. An age-level score is obtained for the three developmental categories; also computed are an overall mean age and a developmental quotient. The profile is designed for use with children from birth to 6 years of age.

Test Name: *Milani-Comparetti Developmental Scale* (1973)
Author(s): A. Milani-Comparetti and E. A. Gidoni
Publisher: Meyer Children's Rehabilitation Institute
Address: University of Nebraska Medical Center, Omaha, NE 68131

Purpose/Description: The *Milani-Comparetti Developmental Scale* is a series of simple procedures designed to evaluate a child's physical development from birth to about 2 years. By using this test, a physician, therapist, or public health nurse can determine in a short period whether a child's physical development corresponds to that of a normal child's. The individually administered procedures are divided into two parts. The first half of the test evaluates the child's motor development. This series of procedures is called spontaneous behavior and assesses the child's ability to control the head and body, to move from one position to another, to stand up from a supine position, and to move about. It consists of nine procedures. The second half of the test asseses those reactions that are predictable — that is, those responses that a normal child automatically gives to specific stimuli. These responses appear in the normal child at fairly specific times in the child's development. This portion of the test is called evoked responses and consists of 18 different procedures. One characteristic of the Milani-Comparetti test is its simplicity. The test can be administered on a table with no special equipment. It may also be administered repeatedly. Repeated evaluations are often valuable as they assist in the detection of developmental delay. The test is not a substitute for standardized tests of infant behavior. Rather, it is a complement to such instruments. It is intended to be used with children from birth to 2 years.

Test Name: *Miller Assessment for Preschoolers* (MAP) (1982)
Author(s): L. J. Miller
Publisher: Kid Technology
Address: 11715 E. 51st Avenue, Denver, CO 80239

Purpose/Description: The MAP was developed to provide a statistically sound, short screening tool that could be used to identify children who exhibit moderate preacademic problems affecting one or more areas of development. In addition, it was developed to provide a comprehensive, structured clinical framework that would be helpful in defining strengths and weaknesses and would indicate possible avenues of remediation. It is an individually administered screening tool that provides a comprehensive overview of a child's developmental status with respect to other children the same age. Twenty-seven core items make up the MAP, but it is designed to be given as a unit only. The score is valued only if based on performance of all the test items. The items can be grouped as follows:

1. Sensory and motor abilities: Sense of position and movement, sense of touch, basic components of movement and coordination.
2. Cognitive abilities: Verbal and nonverbal items examining memory, sequencing, comprehension, association, and expression.
3. Combined abilities: Items requiring the interpretation of visual-spatial information.

The kit includes an examiner's manual, cue sheets, item score sheet and behavior during testing, record booklet, drawing booklet, scoring transparency, and scoring notebook. The materials are contained in a carrying case that also provides a shield, enabling the examiner to prepare test materials out of view of the child. The MAP is intended for use with children 2 years, 9 months, to 5 years, 8 months.

Test Name: *Minnesota Child Development Inventory* (MCDI) (1972)
Author(s): H. Ireton and E. Thwing
Publisher: Behavior Science Systems, Inc.
Address: P.O. Box 1108, Minneapolis, MN 55440

Purpose/Description: The MCDI was devised to furnish pediatricians and other clinicians working with school-age children with a means of evaluating a child's development without the expenditure of professional time. The MCDI is a standardized instrument that uses the mother's observations to measure the development of her child. The inventory consists of a booklet and an answer sheet for the mother and a profile deduced from her replies. The booklet contains 320 statements that describe the behaviors of children in the first 6½ years of life. These statements were selected on the basis of (1) representation of real developmental skills, (2) observability by mothers in real life situations, (3) descriptive clarity, and (4) age-discriminating power. The mother indicates those statements referable to her child's behavior by marking yes or no on the answer sheet. The 320 items have been grouped into eight scales: general development, gross motor, fine motor, expressive language, comprehension-conceptual, situation comprehension, self-help, and personal social. The MCDI can be completed for children ranging in age from 6 months to 6 years. There is limited room for growth at the top of the inventory; it would be difficult to demonstrate a range of skills for children at the upper end of the age range.

Test Name: *Minnesota Infant Development Inventory* (MIDI) (1980)
Author(s): H. Ireton and E. Thwing
Publisher: Behavior Science Systems, Inc.
Address: P.O. Box 1108, Minneapolis, MN 55440

Purpose/Description: The MIDI was designed to obtain and summarize a mother's observations of her baby's current development. It measures development in five areas: gross motor, fine motor, language, comprehension, and personal-social. It provides an opportunity for the mother to describe her baby and report any problems or concerns about the child. The inventory consists of a test booklet of 75 statements that describe the developmental behaviors of children in the first 15 months of life. This is an individually administered instrument. It is designed for children ranging from 1 to 15 months.

Test Name: *A Motor Development Checklist* (1976)
Author(s): A. M. Doudlah
Publisher: Library Information Center
Address: Central Wisconsin Center for the Developmentally Disabled, 317 Knutson Drive, Madison, WI 53704

Purpose/Description: The purpose of the checklist is to assess the child's motor development in terms of spontaneous action patterns, which are stated to be the most representative of a child's status. The sequence of motor development can be used for planning and evaluating the effectiveness of therapy programs. The sequence of motor development is considered crucial; time and rate of development are not as important. The checklist is an observational record and consists of a videotape, Motor Development Checklist, and scoresheets. Observation is done monthly, and length of observation depends on the spontaneous motor movements of the child. The scoring can be done in two ways: (1) by indicating the presence of motor behavior or (2) by using the following scale: does not perform task, beginning to attempt task, performs task occasionally, or performs task skillfully. The second scoring method provides more time-related information about progress. The profile is for use with children from birth to the walking state (approximately 15 months).

Test Name: *Observation of Communicative Interaction* (OCI) (1986)
Author(s): M. Klein and M. Briggs
Publisher: California State University
Address: 5151 State University Drive, Los Angeles, CA 90032

Purpose/Description: The OCI has been developed for use as an informal observation guide to assist in describing the interaction strategies used by parents. It is intended for use as a clinical observation tool. The OCI is administered during an observation in which the caregiver is involved in a routine interaction with the infant. It may be administered with or without the caregiver's awareness.

Test Name: *Portage Guide to Early Education* (rev.) (1976)
Author(s): S. Bluma, M. Shearer, A. Frohman, and J. Hilliard
Publisher: The Portage Guide
Address: Cooperative Educational Service Agency 12, 412 East Slifer Street, Portage, WI 53901

Purpose/Description: The Portage guide (rev.) was developed to serve as a guide to those who need to assess a child's behavior and plan realistic curriculum goals that lead to additional skills. The checklist and card file can aid in assessing present behavior, targeting emerging behavior, and providing suggested techniques to teach each behavior. The guide contains three parts: (1) a checklist of behaviors on which to record an individual child's developmental progress, (2) a card file listing possible methods of teaching those behaviors, and (3) a manual of directions for using the checklist and card file and methods for implementing activities. The checklist serves as a method of informal assessment. The checklist is color-coded and divided into six developmental areas: infant stimulation, socialization, language, self-help, cognitive, and motor. A checklist can be completed on each child on entry into a program. The checklist can serve as an ongoing curriculum record for all of the preschool years; essentially, the same checklist can be used each year. The behaviors are listed sequentially, at one-year intervals, for each category from birth to 6 years. The guide is designed to be a curriculum planning tool. The information derived from it is used to delineate those skills acquired and those yet to be taught. The skills listed on the checklist are behaviorally stated. No specific criteria are provided, although some items do include examples. The examiner might refer to the card file to determine specific activities that could be used to assess the skill. There is a total of 580 items (535 if the infant stimulation items are not used). The checklist as well as the entire Portage guide can be used with children between the mental ages of birth and 6 years of age; the materials can be used with normal preschool children or preschool children with handicaps.

Test Name: *Preschool Attainment Record* (PAR) (research ed.) (1966)
Author(s): E. A. Doll
Publisher: American Guidance Service
Address: Publisher's Building, Circle Pines, MN 55014

Purpose/Description: The PAR is an expansion of the early age levels of the Vineland Social Maturity Scale and is designed to measure the physical, social, mental, and language attainments of young children. This individually administered record includes eight categories of development: ambulation, manipulation, rapport, communication, responsibility, information, ideation, and creativity. For each category there is one item per 6-month age interval. Item types, arrangement, and standardized interview procedures are the same as those of the Vineland Social Maturity Scale. The appraisal is conducted by an interview and observations. The record can be used with children ranging in age from birth to 7 years. It is well adapted for testing deaf, blind, or aphasic children; children with cerebral palsy, mental retardation, autism, or schizophrenia; and children whose development has been impaired by sensory or cultural deprivation or who do not speak English.

Test Name: *Preschool Language Scale* (1969)
Author(s): I. L. Zimmerman, V. G. Steiner, and R. L. Evatt
Publisher: Charles E. Merrill Publishing Co.
Address: 1300 Alum Creek Drive, Columbus, OH 43216

Purpose/Description: The *Preschool Language Scale* was designed to detect language strengths and deficiencies. It consists of two main sec-

tions: auditory comprehension and verbal ability. A supplementary articulation section is also included. Test materials include a manual, picture
book, and 16-page test scale form. The auditory comprehension scale
consists of subtests that require a nonverbal response such as pointing to
a picture the examiner has named. The verbal ability scale consists of
items that require a child to name or explain. The articulation section
requires the child to say words and sentences after the examiner. The
scale is not a test but an evaluation instrument, still in experimental
form, to be used to detect language strengths and weaknesses. The scale
can be used with children from 18 months to 7 years. The authors claim
that it can be used with children of all ages who are assumed to be
functioning at a preschool or primary language level.

Test Name: *Receptive-Expressive Emergent Language Scale*
Author(s): K. Bzoch and R. League
Publisher: PRO-ED
Address: 8700 Shoal Creek Boulevard, Austin, TX

Purpose/Description: The purpose of the REEL is to identify very young
children who may have specific handicaps requiring early habilitative
and educational intervention. The REEL scale is administered principally
through a parent or informant inteview. The instructions allow considerable license in probing for information on each item. The manual recommends but does not require direct observation of the child to confirm
questionable parent responses. Beginning with the startle response
(birth to 1 month), the test extends to a 36-month level. Six items (three
expressive, three receptive) are listed for each one-month interval
through the first year. The second year items span two-month intervals;
the third year, three-month intervals. The scale is founded on two basic
premises regarding language function: (1) the auditory modality is the
primary means of acquiring language and (2) speech behavior and cognition are inseparably interconnected. The REEL scale is intended for use
with children from birth to 36 months.

Test Name: *Reflex Testing Methods for Evaluating CNS Development* (2nd
ed.) (1979)
Author(s): M. R. Fiorentino
Publisher: Charles C Thomas
Address: 301-327 East Lawrence Avenue, Springfield, IL 62717 (217)
789-8980

Purpose/Description: The purpose of the test is to determine neurophysiologic reflexive maturation of the CNS at the spinal, brain stem,
mid-brain, and cortical levels. The manual presents a normative sequen-

tial development of reflexive maturation and possible abnormal responses found in individuals with CNS disorders, such as cerebral palsy. Photographs and explanations of reflex responses and test positions with normal and abnormal responses are illustrated. Each reflex tested can be rated on a reflex chart and resulting functional responses on a motor development chart. Testing takes approximately 20 to 30 minutes. The test can be administered to children from birth through 6 years.

Test Name: *Rockford Infant Developmental Evaluation Scales* (RIDES) (1979)
Author(s): Project RHISE, Children's Development Center
Publisher: Scholastic Testing Service
Address: 480 Meyer Road, Bensenville, IL 60106

Purpose/Description: The RIDES provides an informal indication of a child's developmental status in five major skill areas. The RIDES checklist consists of 308 developmental behaviors for ages ranging from birth to 4 years. They represent the most commonly cited descriptors of normal development found in the professional literature. Items are placed within age ranges and skill areas. The five skill areas are personal-social-self-help, fine motor/adaptive, receptive language, expressive language, and gross motor. The RIDES is designed for use with children from birth to 4 years of age.

Test Name: *Scales of Independent Behavior* (SIB)
Author(s): R. H. Bruinicks, R. W. Woodcock, R. F. Weatherman, and B. K. Hill
Publisher: DLM Teaching Resources
Address: One DLM Park, P.O. Box 4000, Allen, TX 75002

Purpose/Description: The SIB is designed to assess behaviors needed to function independently in home, social, and community settings. This individually administered test consists of four adaptive behavior clusters that include two to five subscales. They are as follows:

1. Motor skills cluster: Gross motor, fine motor
2. Social and communication skills cluster: Social interaction, language comprehension, and language expression
3. Personal living skills cluster: dating and meal preparation, toileting, dressing, personal self-care, and domestic skills
4. Community living skills cluster: Time and punctuality, money and value, work skills, and home-community orientation.

The broad independence cluster (full scale) is a measure of independence based on the results of all 14 subscales. A short-form scale provides a brief measure of broad independence and the early development scale provides a developmental measure of adaptive behavior from infancy to 3 years. The manual recommends allowing one hour for administering the full scale and 15 minutes for the other options. Norms are provided for infants to adults (over 40 years). The early development scale allows the test to be used with infants and severely retarded individuals developmentally 2½ years or younger.

Test Name: *Sequenced Inventory of Communication Development* (SICD) (1975)
Author(s): D. L. Hedrick, E. M. Prather, and A. R. Tobin
Publisher: Western Psychological Services
Address: 12031 Wilshire Boulevard, Los Angeles, CA 90023

Purpose/Description: The SICD attempts to assess systematically receptive and expressive communication development for children aged 4 months to 4 years. The ultimate purpose is to increase efficiency for remedial programming both in the home and in the educational setting. There are two major sections to the inventory: a receptive scale and an expressive scale. The factors assessed in the receptive scale are awareness, discrimination, and understanding. The expressive scale is intended to represent a cross-section of linguistic and psychological paradigms. Five factors are presented. Three represent communicative behaviors: initiating, imitating, and responding behaviors. Two represent linguistic behaviors: verbal output and articulation. The initiating, imitating, and responding behaviors are further subdivided into three assumed levels of progression: motor response, vocal response, and verbal response. The items include a developmental range from 4 to 48 months.

Test Name: *Stanford-Binet Intelligence Scale,* Form L-M, (1916, 1937, 1960, 1973)
Author(s): L. M. Terman and M. A. Merrill
Publisher: Riverside Publishing Co.
Address: 1919 South Highland Avenue, Lombard, IL 60148

Purpose/Description: The *Stanford-Binet Intelligence Scale* assesses general intellectual ability. The authors emphasize that it is not suited to the measurement of differential aptitudes. The Stanford-Binet is an individually administered intelligence test that can be given to individuals from age 2 years up through adulthood. All materials required for administering the test are included in a compact carrying case. Materials appear to be adequate in terms of their size, durability, and usefulness for a wide range. The picture materials are, for the most part, black and white line drawings. These drawings are clearly presented; they may have somewhat limited appeal for very young children, who often respond more readily to colored illustrations. The manual for administering the test is included in the carrying case. The Stanford-Binet can be administered to individuals ranging in age from 2 years to 18 years (adulthood).

Test Name: *Uniform Performance Assessment System* (UPAS) (1981)
Author(s): N. G. Haring, O. R. While, E. B. Edgar, J. Q. Afflick, and A. H. Hayden
Publisher: Charles E. Merrill Publishing Co.
Address: 1300 Alum Creek Drive, Columbus, OH 43216

Purpose/Description: The UPAS is an instrument designed to monitor the progress of individuals whose skills are normally acquired between birth and the sixth year. UPAS was developed specifically to assist teachers and parents in meeting the needs of handicapped individuals. UPAS is a curriculum-referenced test that helps teachers and parents select which skills and behavior should be targeted for instructions for young or low-functioning pupils. There are four major curricular areas addressed by UPAS and organized in separate sections: (1) preacademic/fine motor development, (2) communication, (3) social/self-help skills, and (4) gross motor development. An additional section focuses on specific problems dealing with inappropriate behaviors. The UPAS has approximately 250 items with between 45 and 76 items on a given subscale. The UPAS tutor needs to have the UPAS criterion tests manual, UPAS stimulation cards, and UPAS records forms to complete an assessment. The criterion tests manual describes each test item and how it should be assessed. Each criterion test defines skills in terms that are observed directly and easily tested and describes specific standards for acceptable performance. The criterion tests are labeled according to curricula area and item number within each of the four aforementioned areas. The skill needed, equipment and materials, test/observation procedure, and criteria for scoring are included on each criterion test card. The UPAS is designed for children from birth to 6 years.

Test Name: *Verbal Language Development Scale* (VLDS) (1971)
Author(s): M. Mecham
Publisher: American Guidance Service
Address: Publisher's Building, Circle Pines, MN 55014

Purpose/Description: The author developed this informant-interview scale of verbal language development as a method of assessing what a child does in daily life communicative activities. The VLDS is an extension of the communication portion of the Vineland Social Maturity Scale. The instrument is a 50-item scale that is designed to be administered to an informant regarding the child's performance on tasks that are primarily verbal. The 50 items serve as a basis for obtaining language age equivalents. The scale is purported to be used with children ranging in age from birth to 15 years. It is interesting to note, however, that 37 items reflect child behavior before 6½ years; only 5 items reflect child behavior for ages 9 to 15 years.

Test Name: *Vineland Adaptive Behavior Scales*
Author(s): S. S. Sparrow, D. S. Balla, and D. V. Cicchetti
Publisher: American Guidance Service
Address: Publisher's Building, Circle Pines, MN 55014

Purpose/Description: The *Vineland Adaptive Behavior Scale* is a revision of the Vineland Social Maturity Scale (Doll, 1965). It is intended to assess an individual's performance of the daily activities required for personal and social self-sufficiency. The scales measure adaptive behavior in four domains: communication, daily living skills, socialization, and motor skills. There are three versions of the revised Vineland: (1) The interview edition — survey form, which includes 297 items and provides a general assessment of adaptive behavior, (2) the interview edition — expanded form, which includes 577 items and offers a more comprehensive assessment of adaptive behavior in addition to a systematic basis for preparing individual educational, habilitative, or treatment programs, and (3) the classroom edition, which includes 244 items and assesses adaptive behavior in the classroom. The scales are individually administered to a respondent (parent or caregiver, or classroom teacher) who is familiar with the daily activities of the individual being assessed. The *Vineland Adaptive Behavior Scale* is applicable for all ages. The survey form and expanded form assess individuals from birth to 18 years, 11 months of age, and low functioning adults. The classroom edition is appropriate for students 3 to 12 years, 11 months.

Test Name: *Vocabulary Comprehension Scale* (1975)
Author(s): T. E. Bangs
Publisher: Teaching Resources
Address: 50 Pond Park Road, Hingham, MA 02043-4382

Purpose/Description: The purpose of the *Vocabulary Comprehension Scale* is to provide teachers of language or learning handicapped children with baseline information related to comprehension of pronouns and words of position, quality, quantity, and size. The author suggests that this baseline data will enable the teacher to plan classroom and home activities that will assist the child in developing a vocabulary that will be appropriate for entrance into kindergarten or first grade. The scale consists of 61 items. Objects rather than pictures are used, as the author felt this would increase the reliability of responses. Most of the words, except for the pronouns, are paired opposites. Materials are provided to develop two different scenes for eliciting responses from the children. A tea set and a male and female doll are used to measure the child's comprehension of pronouns. A garage with trees, a fence, a ladder, cats, and a dog are used to elicit responses for most of the words of position, quality, quantity, and size. A few additional items are provided to measure the comprehension of words not included in the two scenes. All items are administered according to the directions on the scoring form. The child is asked to name or point to all the objects before beginning the actual assessment. The items are arranged according to four categories: garage scene, tea party scene, buttons, and miscellaneous. The scale was standardized on a population of children ranging in age from 2 to 12 years.

Test Name: *Vulpe Assessment Battery* (VAB) (1969, rev. 1979)
Author(s): S. G. Vulpe, E. I. Pollins, and J. Wilson
Publisher: Canadian Association for the Mentally Retarded
Address: Kinsmen NIMR Building, York University Campus, 4700 Keele Street, Downsview (Toronto), Ontario, Canada M3J 1P3, (416) 661-9611

Purpose/Description: The purpose of the VAB is to provide a test of competencies in various developmental areas and to provide a sequential teaching approach. The *Vulpe Assessment Battery* is an individually administered comprehensive test including items/activities in the areas of: (1) basic senses, developmental reflexes, postural mobility, balance, motor planning, and muscle strength; (2) environment (physical plan and caregiving personnel); (3) organizational behaviors, attention, motivation, response to environmental limits, dependence, independence; as well as the usual areas of gross motor, fine motor, expressive language, receptive language, and activity of daily living. There are many suggestions under each of these areas. There is a total of 1,340 possible items on the test. The battery was designed for children developing atypically from birth through 6 years of age.

Test Name: *Wechsler Preschool and Primary Scale of Intelligence* (WPPSI) (1967)
Author(s): D. Wechsler
Publisher: The Psychological Corporation
Address: 7555 Caldwell Avenue, Chicago, IL 60648

Purpose/Description: The WPPSI provides a systematic appraisal that purports to measure the mental ability of young children. It continues the theoretical and methodologic approaches to the measurement of mental ability that were the principles used in the construction of the Wechsler Intelligence Scale for Children (WISC). The WPPSI is actually a downward extension of the Wechsler Adult Intelligence Scale (WAIS) and the WISC. The WPPSI consists of a battery of subtests, each of which, when treated separately, may be considered as measuring a different ability and when combined into a composite score may be considered a measure of overall or global intellectual capacity. It consists of 11 subtests, six verbal (one is optional) and five performance. Eight of the subtests are similar to subtests of the WISC, although there are modifications. The directions for administering and scoring the WPPSI are clearly contained in the test manual. The materials are durable and not ambiguous. Examiners trained in the process of individual test administrations and psychology should have no trouble administering and interpreting the WPPSI. The WPPSI has been developed for use primarily with children 4 to 6½ years old. In general, the authors recommend that the WPPSI be used instead of the WISC at levels where the two scales overlap.

Test Name: *Woodstock-Johnson Psycho-Educational Battery* (WJPEB) (Parts 1–3, 1977; Part 4, 1984)
Author(s): R. W. Woodcock, M. B. Johnson, R. H. Bruininks (Parts 1–3); R. F. Weatherman and B. K. Hill (Part 4)
Publisher: DLM Teaching Resources
Address: P.O. Box 4000, One DLM Park, Allen, TX 75002

Purpose/Description: The WJPED is a wide-range comprehensive set of tests for measuring cognitive ability, achievement, interests, and independent behavior. The authors state that the battery was designed as an overview rather than as a tool for in-depth diagnosis. This individually administered battery is organized into four parts. Part 1 is intended to provide information regarding a subject's cognitive functions and scholastic achievements: reading, mathematics, written language, science, social studies, and humanities. Part 3 measures a subject's level of preference for participating in various scholastic and nonscholastic forms of activity. Part 4 is intended to provide information regarding an individual's functional independence and adaptive behavior in motor skills, social and communicative skills, personal living skills, and communicating living skills. Norms are provided for the preschool (age 3 years) to the geriatric (age 80 years) level.

Index

Accidents, 46, 49-50
Accreditation, 56
Adolescent pregnancy, 41-42, 49
AGA (appropriate for gestational age infants), 34
Age
  to initiate assessment, 102-104
  of initiation of service, 14-15
  language comprehension and, 167
  maternal
    Down syndrome and, 31-32
    infant mortality risk and, 49
    low birth weight and, 41-42
Albert Einstein Neonatal Neurobehavioral Scale Manual, 175
Alcohol abuse, maternal, 42
Allied health professional, 56
American Occupational Therapy Association (AOTA), 73
American Physical Therapy Association (APTA), 72
Anticonvulsants, 43
AOTA (American Occupational Therapy Association), 73
Apgar scale, 174, 175
Appropriate for gestational age infants (AGA), 34
APTA (American Physical Therapy Association), 72
Assessing Linguistic Behaviors Scale, 166
Assessing Prelinguistic and Early Linguistic Behaviors in Young Children test battery, 159
Assessment, infant-toddler. *See also* Family assessment
  components of, 64
  data collection strategies
    direct testing, 93
    formal observations, 92
    informal observations, 92-93
    medical personnel reports, 94-95
    parental report, 93-94
    teacher report, 94
  definition of, 92
  developmental domains of. *See specific developmental domains*

early detection of developmental pathology, 89
early intervention programs and, 57
general considerations, 88-92
  decision on appropriate intervention, 89-90
  monitoring of family and child change, 90
  monitoring of program effectiveness, 90-91
  predictive ability of developmental tests, 95-96
  predictive purposes, 91-92
  viewing assessment results, 96-97
intervals, 104-106
limitations of, 103
methodology in, 111
model systems
  in Iowa, 82-83
  in Maryland, 83
  in Massachusetts, 83
  in New Jersey, 83
  in Texas, 84
models for early casefinding, 79-81
P.L. 99-457 and, 20
professionals in, 69-70
  audiologist, 74
  early childhood education specialist, 78-79
  nurse, 75-76
  occupational therapist, 72-73
  physical therapist, 71-72
  physician, 70-71
  psychologist, 76-77
  social worker, 77-78
  speech-language pathologist, 74-75
rationale for, 88-89
recipients of, 26-50
settings for
  center-based, 68-69
  home, 66-68
specific considerations
  assessment intervals, 104-106
  for atypical infants and toddlers, 110-111
  corrections for prematurity, 97-99

Assessment, infant-toddler, specific
considerations — *Continued*
determination of infant state,
106–110
need for serial assessment,
101–102
significance of catch-up growth,
99–101
when to initiate assessment
activity, 102–104
Assessment instruments. *See also*
specific assessment instruments
for cognitive domain, 185–188
criterion-referenced, 132, 133
domain-specific, 130
global, 129
norm-referenced, 130–131, 133
types of, 128
Assessment of Preterm Infants'
Behavior test, 175
Assessment services, enhancement of,
222–230
Assessment strategies, new and
innovative, 229
Attachment
definition of, 148–149
maternal, 148–150
Audiologist, 74, 75
Audiology
interdisciplinary issues, 217
training and curricula needs, 216
Auditory behavior, developmental, 112
Auditory brainstem response testing, 74
Auditory stimuli, aberrant responses
to, 112

Babinski response, 178
Bayley Scales of Infant Development
auditory behavior, developmental, 112
domains of, 131
global assessment and, 129
language expression and, 172
manner of response and, 109–110
for mental development assessment,
186
motor functioning, 181–182
problem solving and, 112–113
vocabulary checklist tasks and, 163
Behavior modification, 7–8
Behavioral organization, stages of, 107
Behaviors, gesture inventory, 158–161
Birth weight, low, 33–39
Blacks, infant mortality rate of, 49

BNBAS (Brazelton Neonatal Behavioral
Assessment Scale), 174–175
Brain damage, 96
Brazelton Neonatal Behavioral
Assessment Scale (BNBAS),
174–175
Brown University infant specialist
degree program, 213, 214
Brown vs. Board of Education, 3–4

Caregiving, deficiencies in, 149
Carolina Institute for Research on
Infant Personnel Preparation,
211–213
working conference of, 213–220
Case history information, obtaining,
120–125
Case management
resource linkage and, 191
services of, 17
system of, 57, 65–66
Case manager, function of, 65
Catch-up growth, 99–101
Center-based assessment, 68–69
Central nervous system organization,
175
Cerebral palsy, 36, 180
Certification
of audiologist, 75
of early childhood education
specialist, 79
of nurses, 76
of occupational therapist, 73
of physician, 71
of psychologist, 77
of social worker, 78
of speech-language pathologist, 75
team approach to health care and,
56–57
Child change, monitoring of, 90
Child find systems, statewide, 224
Children
aged 3 through 5. *See* Toddlers
handicapped
rights of, P.L. 94-142 and, 12–13
status of, federal legislation and,
10–11
infants. *See* Infants
research activity on, 5
Children's rights
Civil Rights movement and, 3–4
historical considerations, 2
societal factors, 2

Child's history form, 243-250
Chromosomal abnormalities, 31-32
Cigarette smoking, maternal, 43
Civil Rights movement, children's
    rights and, 3-4
CMV (cytomegalovirus), 44, 49
Cocaine, use during pregnancy, 43-44
Cognition, definition of, 183
Cognitive development
    newborn stage of, 184
    subjectivity stage of, 184
Cognitive domain
    assessment instruments for, 185-188
    development of, 183-184
    summary of assessment, 188
Cognitive performance, 126
Cognitive play, 151
Coming out, 108
Communication, through gestures, 161
Communication and Symbolic
    Behavior Scales (CSBS), 157-158
Communication specialists, 74-75
Communicative skills, of infants and
    toddlers, 156-157
Comprehension, language, 161-167
Contractual arrangements, 227
Coping ability, of family, 190
Cost-effectiveness, of early
    intervention, 9
Criterion-referenced tests, 132, 133
Cross-training, 63
Crossed adductor reflex, 178
CSBS (Communication and Symbolic
    Behavior Scales), 157-158
Cytomegalovirus (CMV), 44, 49

Data collection, for case history,
    120-125
DDST. *See* Denver Developmental
    Screening Test
Delayed response, 112
Denver Developmental Screening Test
    (DDST)
    correction for prematurity, 99
    description of, 186-187
    domains of, 125, 126-127
    in Iowa model system, 82
Development, child, principles of, 5-6
Developmental cognitive scores, 126
Developmental delay, definition of, 16, 18
Developmental disability
    definition, state development of,
        223-224

degree and severity of, 190
    family stress and, 190
    visibility of, 190
Developmental disorders
    causation of
        accidents and, 46
        categorization of, 50
        contributing factors of, 31-50
        economic factors, 47-50
        environmental influence and, 28
        genetic endowment and, 28
        inadequate prenatal care, 39-40
        interactional model of, 29
        linear cause-and-effect model,
            27-29
        maternal infections and, 44
        maternal nutrition and, 40-41
        maternal smoking and, 43
        nature vs. nurture controversy
            and, 28-29
        perinatal factors, 33-39
        postnatal environmental factors,
            44-50
        prenatal factors, 33-39
        prospective approach to, 26-27
        retrospective approach to, 26
        sociocultural factors, 47-50
        transactional model of, 29-30
        trauma and, 46
    maternal substance abuse and, 42-44
Developmental log, 132-134
Developmental screening
    benefit of, 127-128
    goal of, 125
    instruments for, 125. *See also*
        specific instruments
Developmental services, 191
Developmental tests
    false assumptions from 111
    score corrections for prematurity,
        97-99
Developmental theory assessment
    approach, 186
Diagnosis, 128
Direct testing, 93
Diseases
    childhood, 44-45
    maternal, 44
Domain-specific assessment
    instruments, 130
Down syndrome, 31-32
Drugs
    illegal, use during pregnancy, 43-44

Drugs — *Continued*
  prescription, use during
    pregnancy, 43

Early childhood education specialist
  certification of, 79
  description of, 78-79
  interdisciplinary issues, 216, 217
Early Childhood Intervention Program
    (ECI), 84
Early childhood special education,
    training and curricula needs,
    216, 217
Early Intervention Developmental
    Profile (EIDP), 159, 161
Early Language Inventory, 166
Early Language Milestone Scale (ELM),
    159, 166
Early Social Communication Scales
    (ESCS), 145-146, 147
Economic factors, developmental
    progress and, 47-50
Education
  early, developmental progress and,
    46-47
  early intervention and, 9-10
  public, 224-225
  undergraduate and graduate
    personnel training, 210-213
Education for All Handicapped
    Children Act (P.L. 94-142), 11-15
Education of the Handicapped
    Amendments of 1986 (P.L.
    99-457), 11-15
Education service mandates, 13-14
Educational services, 191
ELM (Early Language Milestone Scale),
    166
Emotional support, for family, 191
Entity-entity relations stage of
    cognitive development, 184-185
Environment
  developmental disorders and, 28
  of home, as setting for infant-toddler
    assessment, 66-68
  meaningful interaction with, 114-115
Environmental awareness, 113
Environmental experience, desire for,
    113-114
Environmental factors, 96
  postnatal, 44-50
Environmental Language Battery, 166
Environmental Prelanguage Battery, 159

ESCS (Early Social Communication
    Scales), 145-146, 147
Experience, early, quality of related to
    developmental progress, 46-47

Family
  change, monitoring of, 90
  service needs of, 191
Family assessment, 229
  description of, 188-192, 229
  paradigm, 192
  of stress, 197-200
  summary of, 200
Family Inventory of Life Events and
    Changes, 192
Family Inventory of Resources and
    Management, 192
Family Needs Survey, 192, 193-194
Family services, 212
Family status, variables, 198
FAS (fetal alcohol syndrome), 42
Federal initiatives, affecting
    handicapped children, 12
Federal legislation, and status of
    handicapped children, 10-11
Fetal alcohol syndrome (FAS), 42
Financial needs, of family, 191
Folic acid antagonists, 43
Follow-up, longitudinal, 105, 229-230
Future issues, 228-230

Genetic factors, in developmental
    disorders, 28, 31-33
Gesell Developmental Schedules, 131,
    187
Gestures, assessment of, 158-161
Global assessment instruments, 129
GMDS (Griffiths Mental Development
    Scale), 99
Grants, federal, for development of
    programs for handicapped
    children, 13
Griffiths Mental Development Scale
    (GMDS), 99
Growth, catch-up, 99-101

Handgrasp, 178
Health maintenance organizations
    (HMOs), 70
Heroin, use during pregnancy, 43-44
High-risk follow-up program
  eligibility criteria for, 82
  questionnaire for, 251-254

High-risk infants
  categories of, 81
  definition of, 34
Home Observation for Measurement
    in the Environment, 125, 192
Home Observation of the Environment
    Inventory (HOME), 197, 199
Home setting, for infant-toddler
    assessment, 66-68
Hospital, interactional opportunity in,
    144
Hypothyroidism, 32

IBR (infant behavior record), 182
ISCI (Infant Scale of Communicative
    Intent), 170, 171
Identification, early, 89, 221-222
  components of, 84-85
  goals for, 21-22
IEP
  purpose of, 13
  vs. IFSP, 17
IFSP (individualized family services
    plan), 17, 19 91
In-service activities, 225, 227
In-turning, 108
Inborn errors of metabolism, 32-33
Individualized family services plan
    (IFSP), 17, 19, 91
Infant behavior record (IBR), 182
Infant-caregiver interaction, language
    domain and, 143-148
Infant Intelligence Scale, 125
Infant specialist degree programs, 213,
    214
Infant state
  definition of, 106
  determination of, 106-110
Infant Temperament Questionnaire
    (ITQ), 196
Infants
  critically ill, parents of, 149
  handicapped
    definition of, 16
    positive aspects of, 30
  high-risk
    categories of, 81
    definition of, 34
  normal development of, research
    studies on, 5-6
  premature
    concept of infant state, 107

  parents of, unexpected realities
    of, 149
  status of
    historical considerations, 2
    societal factors, 2-3
  vulnerable, categories of, 81
Infections, maternal, developmental
    disorders and, 44
Information
  giving, in case history gathering, 124
  obtaining, in case history gathering,
    122-124
Initiation of assessment, timing of,
    102-104
Initiation of infant-toddler assessment
    services, 220-222
Institutionalization, 3
Intake interview
  giving information, 124
  obtaining information, 122-124
  providing release and support,
    124-125
Intelligence quotient, 126
Intensive care, neonatal survival and,
    35, 38
Interactional model of developmental
    disorders, 29
Interdisciplinary issues, 213-220
  cooperation, support of, 227
  delivery of services, 227
Interdisciplinary model of service
    delivery, 59-61
Interdisciplinary training, 211
Intervention
  appropriate, decision on, 89-90
  early, 89
    cost-effectiveness of, 9
    definition of, 16-17
    education classes and, 9-10
    efficacy of, 11
      parent's role in, 7-10
      problems in, 6-7
      study of, 6-10
      variables in, 6
    efficacy of programs for, 90-91
    family and, 189
    goals for, 21-22
    models for early casefinding, 79-81
    objective of, 21
  strategies, accountability of, 13
Interventions, developments to date, 228
Interviews, direct, for case history
    information, 121-122

Iowa, model for infant-toddler
    assessment, 82–83
IQ, maternal malnutrition and, 40

Kent Infant Development Scale, 131
Kleinfelter's syndrome, 32

Language comprehension tests, 163, 166
Language domain, 142–143
    assessment of, summary of, 173
    assessment of gestures, 158–161
    comprehension, 161–167
    expression, 167–173
    infant-caregiver interaction and,
        143–148
    language sampling, 172–173
    play behavior and, 150–155
    pragmatics and, 155–158
Language expression, 167–173
Language production checklists, 170
Language sampling, 172–173
Lead agency, state, 225, 226
Lead poisoning, 45, 49
Least restrictive environment, 12
Licensure. See Certification
Linear cause-and-effect model, 27–29
Listening skills, for case history
    gathering, 122–123
Longitudinal follow-up, 229–230
Longitudinal Neurobehavioral
    Assessment Procedure for
    Preterm Infants, 175
Low birth-weight infants, 33–39
    adolescent pregnancy and, 41–42
    developmental expectations of
        school-age children and, 35
    risk factors of, 35–37, 39
    socioeconomic status and, 47–48
Low-income families, 49

Manipulative behavior, 114
Manual for Analyzing Free Play
    (MAFP), 152
Maryland, infant-toddler assessment
    model of, 83
Massachusetts, infant-toddler
    assessment model of, 83
Maternal age
    Down syndrome and, 31–32
    infant mortality risk and, 49
    low birth weight and, 41–42
Maternal attachment, 148–150
Maternal-infant observation scale, 150

Maternal infections, 49
Maternal nutrition, developmental
    disorders and, 40
Maternal substance abuse,
    developmental disorders and,
    42–44
McCarthy Scales of Children's Abilities,
    129, 131, 187–188
Media, status of handicapped persons
    and, 4
Medical needs, of family, 191
Medicine
    interdisciplinary issues, 217–218
    training and curricula needs, 216
Meningitis, 44–45
Mental retardation
    birth weight and, 39
    Down syndrome and, 31–32
    metabolic disorders and, 32–33
Miller-Yoder Test of Grammatical
    Comprehension, 166
Minnesota Infant Development
    Inventory, 125
MIPIS (Mother-Infant Play Interaction
    Scale), 147–148
Miscellaneous play, 151
Monitoring, 56
    of child change, 90
    of family change, 90
    of program effectiveness, 90–91
Moro reflex, 177
Mortality, neonatal, 49
Mother-infant interaction
    deficiencies in, 145
    talking, 156
Mother-infant interactions, importance
    of, 145
Mother-Infant Play Interaction Scale
    (MIPIS), 147–148
Mother-infant relationship, 8
Mothers, relationship between
    sensitivity and experiences of
    emotional support, 197
Motor Development Checklist, 182
Motor domain
    acquisition of skills, median age of, 179
    assessment of
        during early infancy, 174–176
        following early infancy, 176–179
        summary of, 182–183
    assessment tools for, 181–182
    categories of complications, 180–181
    environmental interaction and, 174

Motor dysfunction in infancy, 180
Multicompetency movement, 63
Multidisciplinary model, of team
    service delivery, 58-59

Nativist view, 3
Nature vs. nurture controversy, 28-29
Neck righting reflex, 178
Neonatal factors, relationship to later
    developmental performance,
    228-229
Neonatal intensive care, infant survival
    and, 35, 38
Neonatal intensive care unit, 143
Neonatal mortality, 49
  low birth weight and, 37-39
Neonatal Perception Inventories (NPI),
    194-196
Neural tube defects, 33
Neurofibromatosis, 33
Neurologic abnormality, criteria for 40
    weeks, 181
Neurologic optimality, neonatal,
    175-176
Neurological Assessment of Preterm
    and Fullterm Infant Scale, 175
New Jersey, infant-toddler assessment
    model of, 83
Newborn stage, of cognitive
    development, 184
Nonstandard expressive language
    assessment procedures, 169-172
Norm-referenced assessment
    instruments, 130-131, 133
Nurse
  certification of, 76
  description of, 75-76
  interactional opportunity with
    hospitalized neonate, 144
Nursing
  interdisciplinary issues, 218
  training and curricula needs, 216
Nutrition
  interdisciplinary issues, 218
  maternal, developmental disorders
    and, 40
  training and curricula needs, 216

Observation of Communicative
    Interaction (OCI), 145
Observations
  of child's language expression, 169

formal, 92
  informal, 92-93
Occupational therapists, 72-73
Occupational therapy
  interdisciplinary issues, 218-219
  training and curricula needs, 216
OCI (Observation of Communicative
    Interaction), 145
Open-ended instruments, 192

Parachute reflex, 178
Parent-child interaction
  impoverished, developmental
    progress and, 46-47
  maladaptive, assessment of, 192,
    194-197
Parent education, 191
Parental report, 93-94
Parents
  behaviors of, age-related and
    maladaptive, 195
  communication of assessment
    results and, 136-137
  giving information to, 124
  home assessment and, 67
  of premature or critically ill infants,
    unexpected realities of, 149
  questionnaire for, 234-242
  role in early intervention, 7-10
  willingness to participate in
    assessment, 103
Peabody Developmental Motor Scales,
    182
Peabody Picture Vocabulary Test, 131,
    162, 163, 166, 172
Perinatal factors, in developmental
    disorders, 33-39
Personnel
  development of, 225, 227
  performance standards of, 20
  qualifications of, 227
  training issues, survey data, 210-213
Phenylketonuria, 32
Physical therapist
  certification of, 71-72
  description of, in infant-toddler
    assessment, 71-72
Physical therapy
  interdisciplinary issues, 219
  training and curricula needs, 216
Physician, description of, in infant-
    toddler assessment, 70-71
Physiologic stage, 108

Piaget, Jean, 183
Play behavior
    categories of, 151, 153-155
    developmental progression in, 155
    language and, 150-155
    measurement of, 151-152
Poisons, environmental, 45
Posture in horizontal suspension test,
    178
Practitioner
    enhancement of service provision,
        222-230
    initiation of assessment services and,
        221
Pragmatics
    definition of, 155
    language and, 155-158
Prediction, of long-term
        developmental expectations,
        91-92
Predictive ability, of developmental
        tests, 95-96
Premature infants
    concept of infant state, 107
    parents of, unexpected realities of,
        149
Prematurity
    catch-up growth, significance of,
        99-101
    corrections for, 97-99
Prenatal care, inadequate,
        developmental disorders and,
        39-40
Prenatal factors, in developmental
        disorders, 33-39
Preschool incentive grant program,
        17-18
Prescriptive interpretation of
        assessment, 135
Preverbal Communication Schedule
        (PVC), 159
Problem solving, 112-113
Professionals
    communication of assessment
        results and, 137-138
    in infant-toddler assessment, 69-70.
        See also specific professionals
Prognostic interpretation of
        assessment, 135
Prospective studies, 26-27
Psychologist
    certification of, 77
    description of, 76-77

Psychology, interdisciplinary issues, 219
Psychometric methodology approach,
        to cognitive assessment,
        186-187
Public education, 224-225
Public law 99-457
    availability of assessment and,
        220-221
    classroom instruction and, 211
    early intervention and, 59
    family services and, 189
    interdisciplinary issues, 214, 227
    service delivery and, 11, 15-16
    title I: handicapped infants and
        toddlers, 16-17
    title II: handicapped children aged
        3 through 5, 17-19
    title III: discretionary programs,
        19-20
    title IV: miscellaneous, 20-21
Public law 94-142 (Education for All
        Handicapped Children Act),
        11-15

Questionnaire
    for case history information, 120-121
    for child's history, 243-250
    for high-risk follow-up clinic
        program, 251-254
    on language usage, 167
    for parents, 234-242

Race
    incidence of low birth weight and, 36
    infant mortality risk and, 49
Receptive-Expressive Emergent
        Language Scale, 125, 162, 166
Receptive One Word Picture
        Vocabulary Test, 162
Reciprocity, 109
Referrals, 65, 70-71
Reflexes, neonatal, 177-178
Rehospitalization, 39, 144
Research
    on efficacy of early intervention
        problems in, 6-7
        variables in, 6
    increased need for, 228-230
Respite care, 191
Results of assessment
    communication of, 136-138
    interpretation of, 134-136
    prescriptive view of, 96-97

Retrospective studies, 26
Rights, of handicapped persons
  children, 2, 3–4
  impact of media on, 4
  impact of support groups, 4
Rubella, 44

Schedule of Recent Events, 199
Screening instruments, for birth to
    three years of age, 127
Separation of means from ends stage
    of cognitive development, 184
Sequenced Inventory of
    Communication Development,
    131, 162
Serial assessment, 101–102
Service delivery, team concept
  interdisciplinary model of, 59–61
  multidisciplinary model of, 58–59
  transdisciplinary model of, 61–64
Service delivery approach, 56–57
Setting, for initiation of infant-toddler
    assessment services, 221
Seventh Annual Report to Congress on
    the Implementation of the
    Education of the Handicapped
    Act, 14–15
Skills, acquisition for assessment
    services, 223
Small for gestational age infants (SGA),
    34
Smoking, during pregnancy, 43
Social communication, 157
Social factors, parental report and,
    93–94
Social interaction, without
    communication, 158
Social play, 151
Social work
  interdisciplinary issues, 219–220
  specialties of, 78
Social worker, 77–78
Sociocultural factors, developmental
    progress and, 47–50
Specialization programs, 211
Specialized care, 190
Speech and language screening
  comprehension items, 164–165
  expression items, 168
Speech-language pathologist, 74–75
Speech-language pathology
  interdisciplinary issues, 220
  training and curricula needs, 216

Spina bifida, 33
Staffing, 65
Stanford–Binet Intelligence Scale, 131
State government
  child find systems of, 224
  contractual arrangements of, 227
  definition of developmental
    disability, development of,
    223–224
  directory of service delivery
    institutions and practitioners,
    225
  funding, 13
  interagency council, 223
  lead agency of, 225, 226
  rankings on incidence of low birth
    weight, 37
Stimuli, new, desire for, 113–114
Strength of response, 112
Subjectivity stage of cognitive
    development, 184
Support groups, status of handicapped
    persons and, 4
Survival
  birth weight and, 34–35
  days in neonatal intensive care and, 38
  neonatal, 143
  neonatal intensive care and, 35
Symbolic play, categorizing of, 153–154
Symbolic relationships stage of
    cognitive development, 185

Talk, mother-infant, 156
Teacher reports, 94
Teachers, 14
Team concept, of service delivery, 56–57
Team leader, 64
Team management issues, 64–65
Teams
  for infant-toddler assessment,
    leadership of, 64–65
  interdisciplinary, 59–60
Test of Auditory Comprehension of
    Language, 166
Tests, standardized, of language
    expression, 169
Texas, infant-toddler assessment model
    of, 84
Thalidomide, 43
Therapeutic counseling, 191
Toddlers
  handicapped, definition of, 16
  P.L. 99-457 and, 17–19

Toddlers — *Continued*
  positive aspects of handicap, 30
  status of
    historical considerations, 2
    societal factors, 2-3
Tonic neck reflex, 177-178
Touching of infant, during
    convalescence, 144
Toxoplasmosis, 44
Training programs, 213
Transactional model of developmental
    disorders, 29-30
Transdisciplinary model of service
    delivery, 61-65

Transient abnormalities of infancy, 180
Trauma, developmental disorders and,
    46, 49-50
Tuning out, excessive, 112

Uzgiris-Hunt Ordinal Scales of
    Psychological Development, 186

Vocabulary checklists, 163
Vocabulary Comprehension Scale, 162

Warfarin, 43